KU-453-347

the beauty pages

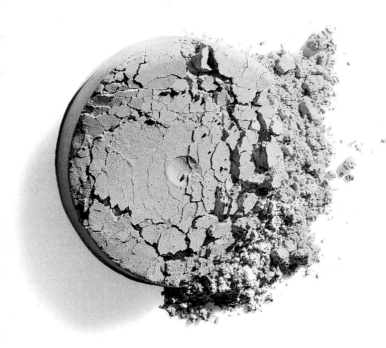

THIS IS A CARLTON BOOK

Text copyright © 2003 Thea Garland
Design copyright © 2003 Carlton Books Limited

This edition published by
Carlton Books Limited 2003
20 Mortimer Street
London W1T 3JW

A CIP catalogue record for this book
is available from the British Library
ISBN 1 84222 753 X
Printed and bound in Singapore

The author and publisher have made every effort to ensure that
all information is correct and up to date at the time of publication.
The application and quality of beauty products and treatments is
beyond the control of the above parties, who cannot be held
responsible for any problems resulting from their use. Always follow
the manufacturer's instructions and, if in doubt, seek further advice.

Note that the product names and prices in this guide are listed for
the UK market and may vary in other countries. If you cannot find the
listed product or price in your country, visit the company's website
(see pages 216–19) for further information. For an idea of the price
conversions for products, please use the simple rate of £1 sterling to
Aus $2.55 and £1 to USA $1.65, accurate at the time of going to press.
Please take into consideration that domestically manufactured products
are usually less expensive than imports.

Editorial Manager: **Judith More**

Art Director: **Penny Stock**

Executive Editor: **Lisa Dyer**

Design: **DW Design**

Copy Editors: **Catherine Bailey, Lara Maiklem
and Libby Willis**

Contributing Writer: **Caroline Jones**

Picture Editor: **Elena Goodinson**

Production Manager: **Lucy Woodhead**

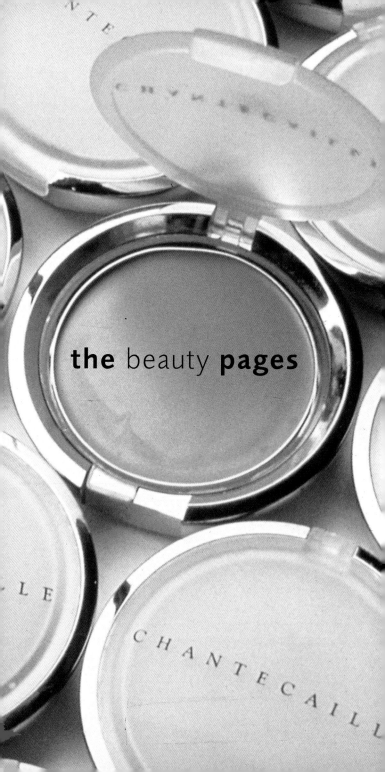

the beauty pages

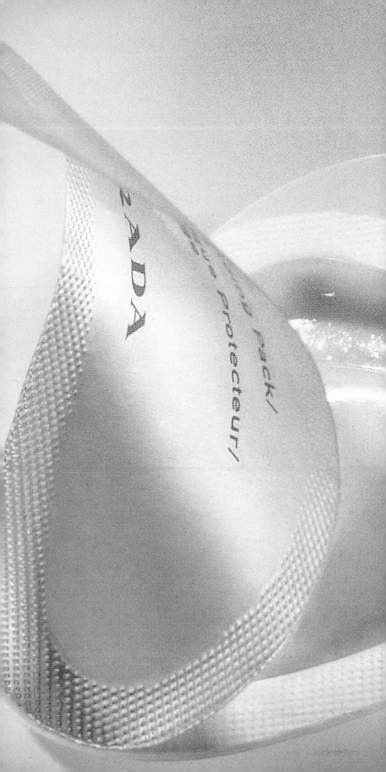

contents

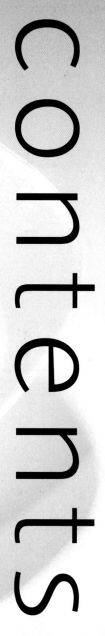

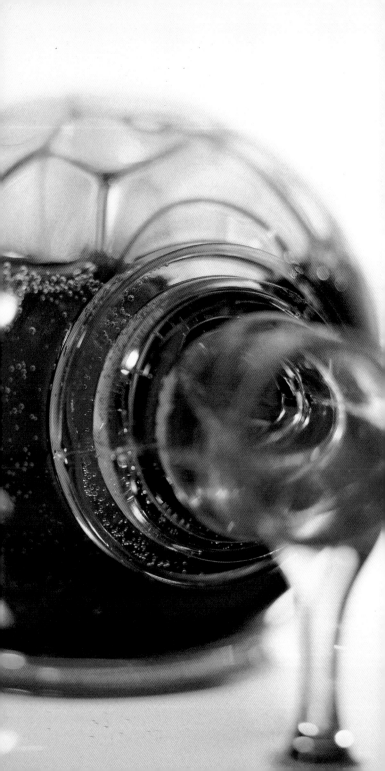

introduction

Beauty has come to represent far more than the pictures we see in glossy magazines or the iconic images in films and on television. Twenty-first century beauty is a form of self-expression; it embraces freedom of style, the ability to make the most of your unique features and to have as much confidence in the way you look as in who you are. The personal care and cosmetics industry has grown by about 5 per cent a year over the past 10 years – that's faster than the world economy. The huge technological advances of the past decade, during which science and skincare have become inextricably linked, have enabled us to slow the ageing process. The skin is able to regenerate itself far more quickly and the appearance of bodily imperfections are dramatically reduced. Products are now versatile, multifunctional and range from the high-tech to the holistic.

The challenge now lies in the choice that is available. In a world where many of us are time deficient, a simple trip to the beauty counter can be a bewildering, even stressful, experience. To be confronted with the sheer number of consumer brands available is overwhelming enough but wading through a plethora of products and deciphering their intended use, translating the technical and chemical terms into common sense language, can be daunting to say the least. Beauty information should be simple, straightforward and practical, so that it is easy to find and buy the products that suit your individual needs and wants. Feeling comfortable and confident in your own skin is 80 per cent of looking beautiful, the remaining 20 per cent should not be a complicated experience.

So, enter this super-friendly consumer guide to find the best buys for you. Designed to fit neatly into your handbag, the book can be easily taken out and referred to on your approach to any beauty counter. Covering every area of beauty – skincare, make-up, haircare and fragrance – and with all entries individually tested, it will tell you which products give the best results. Each of the over 1000 products listed has a review, an explanation of what it is best for and the price and quantity, where applicable. After all, beauty shopping should be fun, so equip yourself... and enjoy!

beauty market news

Trends in the beauty market have become increasingly focused on targeting specific age groups and areas of treatment. Greater interest in well-being, along with the desire for 'double-duty' products, that make you feel as well as look good, has resulted in the emergence of spa-type ranges. Multipurpose items, such as colours that that can be used on the cheeks, eyes and lips, are becoming favourites. As technology continues to progress, sophisticated multifunctional formulas now provide added health benefits as well as pleasure for the senses. Such products include anti-ageing formulas that not only repair existing damage but also slow the ageing process.

Successful global brands, such as L'Oréal, Estée Lauder, and Chanel, have a distinct place in the market, however niche boutique brands are also now emerging as a leading force. Felicity Reilly of the Beyond Beauty buying team at Harvey Nichols, London, says 'consumers are becoming more involved in looking at holistic therapies and traditions to provide solutions to skin problems. But there has also been a parallel interest in the area of cosmeceuticals (see also pages 14–15). Consumers are looking for both prevention and cure, with brands like Dr Hauschka, a range where natural ingredients and holistic production are key factors, and DDF (Doctor's Dermatological Formula), a brand developed by a US dermatologist Dr Howard Sobel.'

Niche brands are often created by personalities with well-founded reputations in the health and beauty fields – Amanda Lacey and Eve Lom skincare products were created by leading facialists and Nars and Laura Mercier cosmetics were created by make-up artists. Influences are also coming from the spa and salon sector, with Bliss Spa launching its own line of products. Some others worth keeping an eye on this year include Z Bigatti, Ole Henriksen and Biotherm.

BRAND IMAGES

Speak to any cosmetic company and they are likely to pride themselves on the quality of their products – including the research, ingredients and the process by which they are made. While this may be true, the image a brand promotes is one of its key selling points. For example, La

Prairie's Swiss skincare range is renowned for its scientific advances that combine anti-ageing cellular therapy with exclusive ingredients. The Christian Dior line, on the other hand, is intrinsically linked to glamour and high fashion, and Aveda markets itself as the most natural brand from the Estée Lauder stable. A brand such as Maybelline will pitch itself as not only being a quality manufacturer but also affordable.

In an industry where a woman's appearance is the highest consideration, aesthetics are paramount, so it is hardly surprising that a significant part of a brand's budget goes into packaging and advertising. One way that brands keep their profile high is to release limited editions. These products have become must-have items, with the company's main line certain to benefit from the exclusivity.

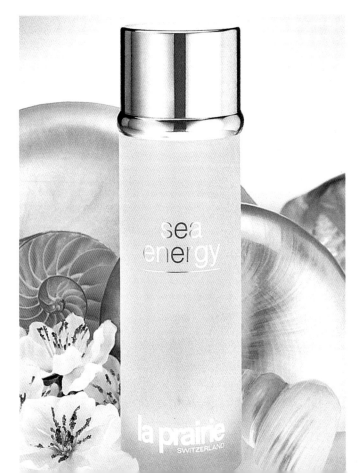

catwalk trends and colour forecasts

Beauty and fashion are intertwined, and the catwalk trends set by couture houses have a strong influence on the make-up we see at the beauty counter. Fashion is cyclical by nature – in continual motion – and each time a new trend appears on the catwalk, beauty will be in step with it. Try to look at trends in context with what is happening for the season. For example, romantic summer clothes may be accompanied by translucent colours or lots of gloss, rather than matt opaques.

Often the amazing-looking make-up that appears on the catwalk is unrealistic and unpractical for a day in the office or at home. And, although cosmetic companies update their colours and products with each season,they always have a classic line available. Seasonal trends are fun and fresh, and can give you a new approach to your make-up, or a new look, but also keep in mind your own needs and what works for you year after year. Investing in just one new colour of eyeshadow or lipstick can allow your look to move with the times. According to Anne Carullow, senior vice-president of global product innovation at Estée Lauder, vibrant and saturated colours – which she calls 'lipstick tones' – will feature throughout winter 2003–2004, and include such hues as lavender, mauve and rose. Tomato reds, poppy and deep corals are also set to make a big impact, while blues – in every tone from cobalt and indigo to periwinkle and grey-blue – will be everywhere. Green shades have also been extended into the winter palette. Dominique Szabo, vice-president of trends at Estée Lauder, says make-up for spring 2004 will be 'extravagant and fun in feminine, happy colours' and that 'you will see refreshing, bright shades for eyes and lips – lush reds, poppies, effervescent, acid-tint yellows and aqua-blues.'

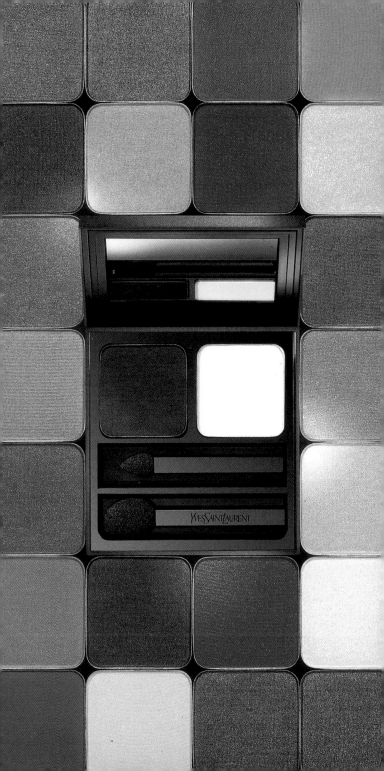

cosmetic labelling

Ingredients on the labels of cosmetics are basically a list of chemicals so, unless you know, for example, that tocopherol is vitamin E and that methylparaben is a synthetic preservative derived from a petroleum base, labels are very often little help.

Regulations require the ingredients to be listed in descending order of quantity. Water is usually found at the beginning of the list while colour, additives and fragrances, usually used in smaller amounts, come at the end. To add to the consumer's confusion, many ingredients have trade names but these rarely provide any clues as to what they are or what they do – there is no way, therefore, of comparing similar ingredients in similar products. Many people, for example, select 'alcohol free' products on the basis that alcohol is said to dry the skin. Alcohols, however, are diverse, with different names and a variety of effects upon the skin. In cosmetic labelling the term 'alcohol' refers to ethyl alcohol, but beware of cosmetics bearing the label 'alcohol free' as they may include it in other forms.

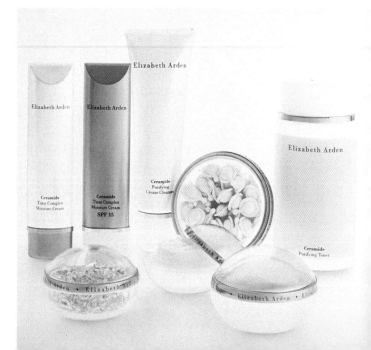

There are no set standards that govern the use of the term
'hypoallergenic'. No cosmetic can be guaranteed to never produce
an allergic reaction, so the term 'non-allergenic' can be misleading.
It is only the list of ingredients that will enable you to detect whether
there is any difference between products that make that claim and
other competing brands. Similarly there are are no legal definitions
for the phrase 'not tested on animals'. In some cases the 'not tested'
can in fact mean not tested at all, but in many cases it means that
companies have simply used ingredients tested on animals by other
companies. Unfortunately the law also does not require cosmetics
manufacturers to substantiate performance claims, so choose carefully.

Below is a brief explanation of the basic terms but for detailed
information see the *International Cosmetic Ingredients Dictionary* and
the other resources listed in the directory (see pages 210–219).

ingredients

Ceramides
Synthetic replicas
of lipids (moisture
molecules) that form
naturally in the skin.
Used in both cleansers
and moisturizers.

DEA
(diethanolamine)
An antioxidant
compound that tightens
and smooths skin
by boosting the
neurotransmitters
within it.

Emollient
Has a moisturizing
effect by holding
water within the skin.

Exfoliant
Removes dead skin
cells, smoothing the
skin and allowing new
cells beneath to absorb
moisturizers better.

Glycerine
A humectant, which
means that it attracts
water moisture from
the air into the skin.

Hydrocortisone
A strong antiseptic that
calms irritated skin and
acne breakouts.

Isopropyl Alcohol
Dissolves ingredients
and colourants into
lotion formulas.

**Para-aminobenzoic
Acid (PABA)**
Used in fake-tan
products, sun blocks
and foundations. Can
cause allergic reactions.

Petroleum Jelly
Seals moisture into skin
with a protective film.

Polysorbates
Stops oil and water from
separating in a formula.

Propylene Glycol
A humectant that helps
to retain moisture. Can
also be a skin irritant.

**Sodium
Lauryl/Laurith
Sulphate**
A detergent and
foaming agent. It can
cause eye irritations,
skin rashes and allergies.

Sorbitol
A humectant that gives
a velvety feel to the skin.
Helps bind moisture
to the skin's surface.

Stearic Acid
When combined with
glycerin, this fatty acid
acts as a humectant.

**Triethanolamine
Stearate**
Used in cleansing
creams to emulsify
oil and water.

cosmeceuticals and treatments

In recent years, the marriage of cosmetics and pharmaceuticals, 'cosmeceuticals', has been the focus of much attention in the beauty and skincare industries. Staggeringly, more than a third of global skincare launches now claim to have cosmeceutical formulations. In fact, by 2006 cosmeceuticals are predicted to be a billion-dollar industry. Just like cosmetics, these serums and bioactive creams are topically applied, but they also contain ingredients, similar to those found in pharmaceuticals, that influence the biological function of the skin. Using naturally derived ingredients, they are usually designed to counteract the effects of sun exposure, free radicals, pollution and ageing. Ingredients include: retinol (a naturally occurring form of vitamin A), vitamin C, vitamin E, Co-enzyme Q10 (a powerful antioxidant and a natural component of human cells), AHAs (alpha-hydroxy acids) and other synthesized molecules and enzymes. Consumers are drawn to cosmeceuticals not only by their claims to slow the ageing process but also because their ingredients are naturally derived. However, 'natural' ingredients can be just as irritating to the skin as artificially synthesized ones. Even a completely natural ingredient is not guaranteed to be reaction-proof.

Drug or cosmetic then? Cosmeceuticals have proved to be rather tricky to label and indeed to retail. The US Food, Drug and Cosmetic Act defines drugs by their intended use; a 'drug' affects the structure or any function of any part of the body, while a 'cosmetic' is deemed to be a product that enhances the appearance of the skin without therapeutic benefit. This means if a claim is made that an antioxidant is able to penetrate beneath the

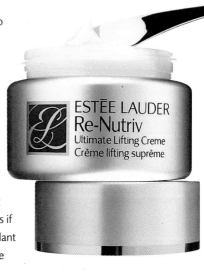

skin's surface in order to remove free radicals, technically it is a drug. The term 'cosmeceutical' has no legal meaning, so the makers of these new-generation products tend to use phrases such as 'reduces fine lines' or 'firming' on the labels. However, some products may be defined as both a cosmetic and a drug, if they have two intended uses. For example, a skin cream that has sun-protection as well as moisturizing properties could fall into this category.

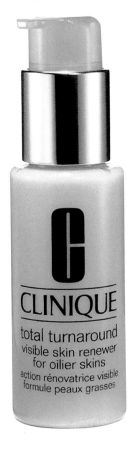

FURTHER ADVANCES

Although AHAs and BHAs (beta-hydroxy acids) have been mainstays for some years, companies are making new forays into the science of skincare. 'Like anything medical, the future of skincare lies in DNA information – it holds the key to the vast amount we don't know,' says Dr Daniel Maes at Estée Lauder. At the Lab 21 counter in Saks Fifth Avenue, New York customers can take a sample of skin cells with diagnostic tape and send it to a lab in Silicon Valley, where the DNA is analyzed and a customized cream is made.

Scientists have also discovered that endorphins can prevent ageing, so these are becoming key ingredients. Clinique's Repairwear includes Vital Fuel, which restores the skin's natural capacity to produce energy, while Guerlain's new Issima Happylogy products contain a complex that helps the skin to create beta-endorphins. Finally a series of muscle-relaxant items are gaining in popularity. Examples include DDF's Wrinkle Relax (originally Faux-Tox) and Givenchy's No Surgetics.

organic and all-natural products

The past decade has seen a surge in the popularity of naturally based products, and a dramatic increase in sales of ranges such as Aveda, Dr Hauschka, Elemis, Jurlique, Liz Earle and Origins. Just as many of us have become more ecologically aware (choosing holistic medicine, organic food and so on), we are now also seeking a natural approach to beauty. When you consider that about 60 per cent of what we put on our skin ends up in our bloodstream, it is hardly surprising. Often the terms 'natural' and 'organic' are overused, and products that might contain only 1 per cent of natural ingredients will display 'all-natural' on their label. Unfortunately, there is no legal definition of what qualifies as 'natural' and as a result, huge discrepancies can arise between brands. Wholesome-sounding ingredients such as honey, strawberry and apple are no guarantee that such products are good for your skin; indeed many of them may go through a lot of harmful processing in order to become cosmetics. In addition, many natural products use many of the same emulsifiers, preservatives and stabilizers as their conventional counterparts to prolong their shelf life.

The Soil Association, the UK's leading organic-certifying body, recently released new health and beauty product standards. To ensure a maximum proportion of organic ingredients, minimum processing and clear labelling, the standards cover the preparation of raw materials through to environmentally-responsible manufacturing. Under these guidelines GM (genetically modified) ingredients are prohibited, and ingredients or processes that have a detrimental environmental effect must also be avoided. Products containing at least 95 per cent organic ingredients can be labelled 'organic' and those with no less than 70 per cent may be labelled as made with a specific percentage. Testing on animals is also prohibited unless required by law, but no guarantee can be made that ingredients haven't been tested on animals in the past – a claim of 'not tested on animals' may not cover all the ingredients.

While chemical products have the advantage of extensive research and testing, they frequently contain preservatives that can cause allergic reactions. Powder-based products such as eyeshadow may contain aluminium, which has been linked to Alzheimer's disease. When opting for a more natural product, you can take steps to avoid ingredients that may cause skin irritations and allergies. Try to avoid anything that contains the following: propylene glycol, paraffin, stearalkonium chloride, isopropyl alcohol, methylisothiazolinone, formaldehyde, sodium laureth sulphate, DEA (diethanolamine) and TES (triethanolamine), and coal tar or synthetic colours (see also page 13).

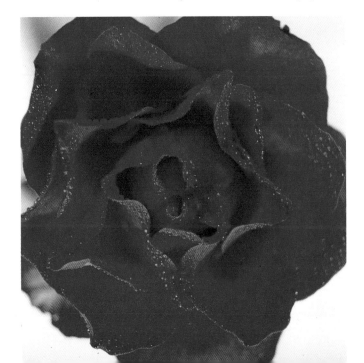

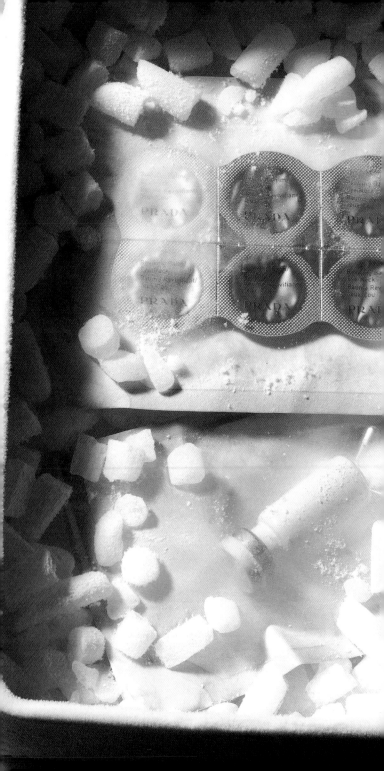

supplements as beauty products

While using the right products will certainly enhance your looks, beauty and health are inseparable. We are what we eat. Just about every beauty guru will say that a healthy diet is vital for gorgeous looks, be it clear skin or cellulite-free legs. However, obtaining adequate nutrition can be difficult as many modern foods are processed and loaded with additives, artificial flavours and colours, and traces of pesticides. As a result, more and more people are taking dietary supplements in the form of multivitamins and minerals.

When choosing a supplement it is important for you to consider your individual needs and to appreciate that good results won't come without healthy eating habits. Vitamins do not provide energy but they are valuable in regulating the metabolism, helping to convert fat and carbohydrates into energy, and assisting the formation of bones and tissue. Though each vitamin has a specific function, they work with one another and with the correct balance of carbohydrates, fats and proteins that is provided by a good diet. They do not fight infections single-handedly but work together in order to maintain the body's natural immune system (see also page 21).

vitamin a: the great anti-ager

One of the great anti-ageing superheroes of our time is vitamin A. Although its derivatives abound on beauty counters, the only term that describes vitamin A in its pure form is retinol.

The birth of this cosmetic wonder-cream began in 1978 when Professor Albert Kligman formulated the prescription drug Retin-A to treat acne. Scientists soon discovered that the drug also stimulated collagen and elastin, reduced fine lines and helped to improve the look of ageing skin. The major drawback with Retin-A was that without proper medical supervision the skin became sensitized, becoming raw and red and vulnerable to damage by sunlight. In spite of this, Retin-A went on to become the prototype for a whole new generation of medical products that were kinder on skin but not benign enough to be sold over the counter.

The next revolutionary event was the release, by cosmetic companies, of a safe form of retinol, available over the counter. This, coupled with the development of an innovative delivery system that allowed active vitamin A to be delivered into the skin, led to the launch of products such as Estée Lauder's Diminish. It is claimed that results are visible after four weeks of use, but retinol products must be used regularly for continual improvement. Retinol users should also wear a high-factor sunscreen as their skin will be more sensitive to UV rays.

Dermatologists suggest that while retinoic acid, as found in prescription drugs such as Retin-A, does help anti-ageing, only concentrations of up to 1 per cent are regarded as safe. Although no categorical proof has been established, there have been reports that Retin-A lotion can result in birth defects when used by pregnant women. So, avoid using Retin-A or other vitamin A derivatives when pregnant, breastfeeding or attempting to become pregnant. Anyone with very sensitive skin should also steer clear of retinol products.

types of vitamin A:

Retinoic Acid
The acid form of vitamin A, which is also known as 'Tretinoin'. The active ingredient in prescription-only products such as Retin-A, Retinova and Retrieve.

Retinol
The pure alcohol form of vitamin A. It is less potent and irritating than retinoic acid and is therefore allowed in cosmetics.

Retinoids
The generic term for all vitamin A derivatives, both naturally occurring and synthetic compounds.

Retinyl palmitate and retinol linoleate
Vitamin A derivatives that are common in many skincare preparations, particularly wrinkle creams and anti-ageing products.

Tazarotene
A relatively new retinoid, previously used in the treatment of acne and psoriasis. It has recently been shown to be beneficial in the treatment of photo-damaged skin.

supplements

Vitamin A

Essential for skin, nails, bones and teeth. Stimulates the growth of skin cells and is used to treat acne. Also an important anti-stress vitamin.

Vitamin B complex

Good for skin and hair. Essential for brain and nervous system health, and improves circulation.

Vitamin C (Ascorbic Acid)

A natural antioxidant and skin protector, essential to the formation of collagen; without it skin becomes bumpy and wrinkled.

Vitamin D

Essential for bone development and prevention of osteoporosis.

Vitamin E

The ultimate skin vitamin – helps heal scar tissue and neutralize damage from free radicals.

Vitamin K

For treating spider veins, broken blood vessels, bruising and even under-eye circles.

Echinacea

Extract of corn flower; strengthens the immune system against infections.

Evening Primrose Oil

Beneficial for skin and hair. Good for alleviating dry skin.

Ginkgo Biloba

Extract of maidenhair tree; good for circulation and varicose veins.

Ginseng

An energy-boosting plant that strengthens the immune system.

Selenium

An antioxidant mineral that is beneficial in the fight against premature ageing.

Spirulina

A blue-green algae that is 60 per cent protein and rich in beta-carotene, vitamin B and minerals. A great energy booster that helps build up the immune system.

Zinc

A protein-rich mineral that is found in every body cell. It stimulates growth and can help to clear spot-prone complexions.

Remember:

- Consult your doctor before beginning a course of dietary supplements.
- Vitamins should be taken during the day. Minerals should be taken at night.
- Vitamins are best absorbed with food or just before a meal.

the a–z of beauty

A is for Antioxidants

Substances (notably vitamins A, C and E and grapeseed extract) that repair the damage to the skin's cells inflicted by free radicals. Free radicals contribute to ageing and are stimulated by factors such as exposure to pollution and ultraviolet light.

B is for Benzoyl Peroxide

An oxygen-releasing chemical included in acne medication that has a drying and antibacterial action on blemishes.

C is for Ceramides

Lipids synthesized to a natural blueprint, ceramides work in the skin's uppermost layer to form a protective barrier between intercellular spaces and reduce moisture loss. A great anti-ageing treatment for dry skin.

D is for Dihydroxyacetone (DHA)

An ingredient used in fake tanning products, which reacts with the skin to provide a sun-tanned appearance.

E is for Eucalyptus Oil

An antiseptic oil with healing properties, it is often included in treatments for problem skin and spa products.

F is for Free Radicals

Unstable molecules that attack body cells, damaging DNA, fats and proteins within them.

G is for Glycolic Acid

Derived from sugar cane, glycolic acid is a potent AHA (alpha-hydroxide acid) and exfoliator. It reduces fine lines and increases skin hydration, but long-term use can leave skin weaker and prone to irritation.

H is for Hyaluronic Acid

Locks essential moisture within the layers of the skin, reducing fine lines.

I is for Iridescence

Make-up products that have the effect of adding glow to the skin and highlighting bone structure.

J is for Jojoba Oil

Derived from the jojoba plant, this natural moisturizer is used in both haircare and skincare products.

K is for Kinetin

Found in green, leafy plants, kinetin is a stable antioxidant that can delay the onset of ageing in skin cells.

L is for Liposome

An ingredient-delivery system with a similar structure and composition to skin cells, liposomes allow active ingredients in skincare products to penetrate into deep layers of the skin.

M is for Microsponges

Microscopic spheres that reduce oiliness and shine by absorbing skin secretions.

N is for Night Cream

Rich moisturizers that penetrate overnight to rehydrate the skin. The new generation contain

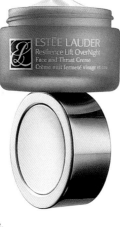

antioxidants to repair damage caused during the day, and some even include relaxing fragrances such as lavender and rose. Although they do smooth and hydrate more mature skins, the jury is still out on whether they are fundamental to skincare.

O is for Oil Control

Oil-control products reduce the excess sebum that can cause breakouts. Anti-blemish solutions and blotting tissues help to reduce a build up of oil, which can be exacerbated by moisturizer and foundation.

P is for Paraffin

Derived from petroleum or coal and found in everything from eyebrow pencils to moisturizers. One ingredient you don't want to see on the label of a product claiming to be 'natural'!

Q is for Co-Enzyme Q-10

Q-10, an enzyme produced naturally in the body that acts as antioxidant, is available as a supplement and in topical preparations.

R is for Rose Water

A gentle alternative to alcohol-based toners, it leaves skin feeling fresh and clean without drying. Ideal for sensitive skins.

S is for Salicylic Acid

A BHA (beta-hydroxy acid) derived from willow bark, this is used in both acne treatments and anti-ageing cosmetics. It helps to 'dissolve' the top layer of skin cells, thereby smoothing the complexion. BHAs are gentler than AHAs, but can still irritate some skin types if used in too high a concentration.

T is for Tea Tree Oil

A plant extract with antiseptic and antibacterial properties, tea tree oil aids healing and treats blemishes.

U is for UVA and UVB Rays

Ultraviolet rays emitted by the sun damage collagen and are responsible for pigmentation and blotchy skin. UVB rays can cause burning, while UVA rays cause ageing because they penetrate deeper to effect long-term damage.

V is for Vitamin B5 (Pro Vitamin B5)

The ultimate beauty vitamin, panthenol stimulates skin healing and provides deep moisturization for both skin and hair.

W is for Witch Hazel

A plant extract with a natural alcohol content of 70 per cent, witch hazel is an astringent and cooling antiseptic.

X is for Exfoliant

Exfoliants buff off dead skin cells, revealing a clearer, fresher complexion.

Y is for Ylang Ylang

A versatile essential oil that has a balancing effect on sebum. It is beneficial for all skin types.

Z is for Zinc

This mineral can help to remedy fatigue and clear problem skin.

choosing products

When selecting a product, it is easy to be confounded by the sheer choice available. Not only is there a huge variety of products available but advertising makes it easy to be swayed by the power of the image, celebrity endorsements and marketing – don't be! There are no hard and fast rules as to which brands work and which don't; it is really a matter of what suits your skin and works for you. Generally the big companies test their products rigorously and it would be difficult, given government regulations, for them to make erroneous claims.

SKIN TYPES

Understanding your skin type will help you choose the best products for your needs. However, given that skin can alter on a day-to-day basis, dependant on internal factors like fluctuations in hormones and stress and external influences such as seasonal changes and pollution levels, it is difficult to classify skin into distinct categories. The information below provides a general guide, but many people find that they need to switch products when their skin changes over the course of the year.

Dry skin With dry skin, sebum production is minimal and pores tend not to be visible. The skin has a propensity to age quickly and can be flaky. Even if your skin is not usually dry, external factors such as wind, central heating and air conditioning can all deplete the skin's supply of moisture. To remedy dry skin, wear a protective moisturizer and invest in a night cream. Cream cleansers are best, and opt for oil-based make-up formulations. Choose cream blushers, which blend effortlessly into skin, rather than powders, which tend to highlight every line.

Oily skin This type of skin secretes a lot of sebum, and while this is an anti-ageing gift – oily skin is usually less affected by external factors – it can also mean open pores and breakouts. Be careful not to overcleanse or use products with a high alcohol content, as this causes sebaceous glands to produce even more sebum. Wash-off cleansers are the best choices, and they leave the skin feeling clean and fresh. Avoid products containing paraffin and lanolin, as these can block pores, and any items

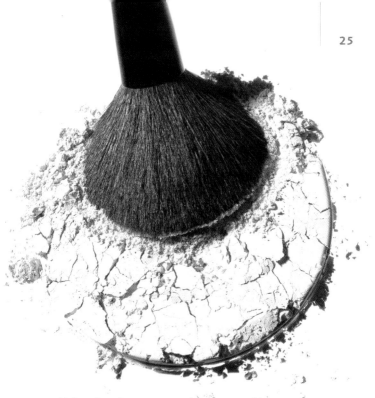

termed 'glossy', as these may contain silicones, which can encourage breakouts. Use a lightweight oil-free moisturizer and an oil-free foundation, and stick to powder blushers and eyeshadows.

Combination skin Skin that possesses both dry and oily components is usually termed 'combination skin'. In people with this type, the T-zone tends to be oilier than that the rest of the face, however the cheeks may experience dryness from time to time. When choosing and applying products, look at your skin – it may be drier in the winter months than in the summer so switching from a wash-off cleanser to a cream cleanser may be necessary. Only moisturize the areas that require moisture.

Sensitive skin Everyone can suffer from an occasional reaction, but genuinely sensitive skin is actually quite rare. If, however, your skin reacts to just about everything, treat it with care: avoid abrasive products, including those with a high alcohol content, artificial scents or surfactants (aggressive cleansers, detergents). Avoid cleansers that contain lanolin, as this can exacerbate flare-ups, and try a mild cream cleanser instead. Look for skin-soothing ingredients such as aloe vera or camomile.

do higher prices mean better quality?

Don't always assume that just because a product costs a small fortune that it is superior to its more affordable counterparts. Read the list of ingredients to see what they both contain, try each, and form your own conclusions. Expensive products will undoubtedly have more luxurious packaging, and often a nicer scent, which gives a positive psychological boost. Major cosmetics companies often produce lower-cost lines in addition to their high-end brands. In these cases the lower-priced versions benefit from the research department of the main company.

what is the shelf life of cosmetics?

Experts tell us that the shelf life of most skincare products is about twelve months. Cleansers, moisturizers and foundations all fall into this category. Lipstick can be used for up to two years, as can powder and eyeshadow, but cosmetics used directly on the eye area should be discarded every three to four months because of the risk of infection. If mascara becomes dry, throw it away; do not add water or oil as this will introduce bacteria into the product. Brushes need to washed every two to three months and sponges should be washed every week and then thrown away after a month. Sun-protection products should be discarded after one year as their active ingredients will begin to lose their protective powers. Other items that are likely to have an unusually short shelf life are certain 'all natural' products, which may contain plant-derived substances conducive to microbial growth. It is also important to take into account the increased risk of

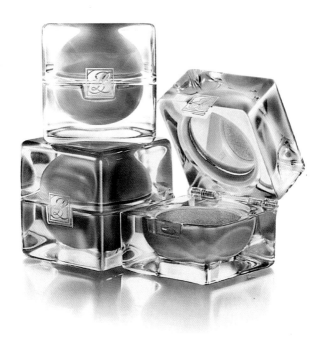

contamination in products that contain non-traditional preservatives, or none at all. 'Expiry dates' are merely a guideline when it comes to determining the longevity. To increase shelf life, store products away from direct sunlight and do not expose them to high temperatures.

applying cosmetics

Luci Rogers, make-up artist for Aveda, says the key to applying make-up lies with accentuating your best assets, whether that is smooth skin, big eyes, luscious lips or shapely brows. Consider your face shape, too. An oval face is the most versatile; therefore shading, bronzing or simply adding a rosy flush are all looks that can be tried. Blusher or bronzer can be applied under the cheekbones to slim down a round face, or around the hairline to slim the top of a heart-shaped face. To slim a heavy jaw, emphasize cheekbones and highlight the eye area. If you are uncertain about shading, then draw attention to either the eyes or the lips.

Make-up artist Ruby Hammer, co-founder of Ruby and Millie cosmetics, advises to avoid perceiving 'flaws' as imperfections but as your own unique features to work with and make the most of. She is a great believer that make-up should be fun, but more importantly it should be specific to your face shape, skin tone and complexion. 'It is vital to look at your skin each morning and evaluate it on a day-to-day basis before applying any sort of make-up. Pick one feature – eyes, lips or cheeks – that you are going to accentuate that day and focus on it alone.' She goes on to say that 'there really aren't any strict rules to abide by when it comes to choosing and applying make-up – the key lies in looking at your skin and basing your decisions around your personal needs, as opposed to following the trends from season to season.' As a general rule, 'less is usually more' and blending is mandatory!

SHOPPING FOR MAKE-UP AND SKINCARE

- Don't be talked into buying products you neither want nor need by salespeople. Write out a list beforehand and stick to it.
- If you are unsure about a product, ask for a sample to try at home before investing in the full size.
- Always test foundation or concealer on your face or neck, and check the colour in natural light before purchasing. Blend several shades along your jawline – the correct one should be invisible!
- Take a mirror in your handbag; this way you will be able to check your foundation in natural light, away from beauty-counter lighting.
- If you have an allergic reaction to a product, take it back! Most cosmetics companies will accept returns under these circumstances.

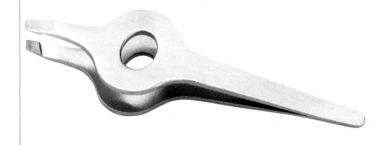

make-up tools

Using the correct tools will make a huge difference to the finished appearance of your make-up.Brushes can be bought from cosmetic companies such Bobbi Brown and Chanel, but also try art stores for great quality brushes at reasonable prices. Your basic brush kit should include the following:

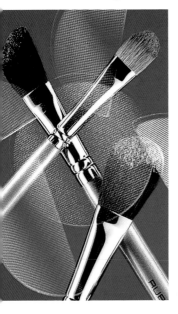

Concealer brush A narrow, short brush (preferably synthetic) for precise coverage of blemishes.
Eyeshadow brush A short, full brush, cut square to glide over lids.
Eyeliner brush Tiny, flat and pointed for drawing fine lines.
Eyebrow brush A brush with reasonably firm, angled bristles.
Blusher brush A medium, full brush, angled to create soft edges.
Powder brush Big, soft and fluffy, this brush gives even coverage of powder or bronzer.
Lip brush Narrow, preferably with natural bristles, for accurate and long-lasting lipstick application.

OTHER VITAL TOOLS:

Tweezers Good-quality, angled metal tweezers are easiest to use.
Powder puff Choose one roughly the same size as your hand. It is essential for creating a smooth, even finish when setting with powder.
Sponge Available in several shapes, these are used to blend in foundation. They need frequent washing.
Eyelash curler Curling your lashes really opens up your eyes, with or without mascara. The metal versions are usually the best performers.
Sharpener If your lip or eye pencils get too blunt you won't be able to draw accurate lines. Invest in a sharpener with two sizes of holes.
Sharp nail scissors Good for all sorts of beauty tasks.

essential make-up kit

Everyone has a different make-up routine and therefore requires products and tools that are specific to their needs for everyday use. The list below includes most of the fundamentals you will need to cover all occasions, but items such as eye drops, petroleum jelly and cotton buds are also useful to have at hand. To extend your basic range, add an extra shade or two of blush, eyeshadow and lip colour.

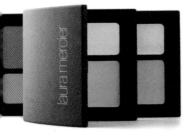

Powder Useful for setting foundation and removing shine during the day, you can choose loose or pressed, although it is good to have one of each – for home and handbag. Make sure that it is as translucent and as invisible as possible, and be aware that powder can look chalky on darker skins.

Concealer Look for a yellow-based concealer with a creamy but non-greasy texture. You should ideally have two concealers: a solid one for covering blemishes and a light-reflective one to soften under-eye shadows and fine lines. Some products are available in several shades for mixing, which is useful if your skin tone changes over the course of the year.

Blusher Pink or peach colours will enhance fairer skin tones, while richer colours look good on dark skins. Subtlety is the key; cream or gel formulas give the most natural effect.

Bronzing powder or cream A bronze-tinted cream or bronzing powder can be used to create a sun-kissed look, and some people opt for a bronzer instead of a blusher. Stay close to your natural skin tone and go for brown rather than orange-toned products, as they look more natural. Bronzing powder can double as a subtle eyeshadow when you're on holiday.

Foundation You may find that you need two shades – one for winter and one for summer – and these can be mixed to create the correct shade for those inbetween times. If you do not like the feel of foundation, you can try a tinted moisturizer.

Eyeshadow Choose shades within the same colour range for a more natural look; you will need a darker tone to apply along the lashline, a medium tone for the socket and the lower part of the eyelid, and a light tone to highlight the browbone. Choose a trio in neutral colours that you will use every day.

Eyeliner Great for defining the eyes, a neutral brown is a useful choice for your basic kit. Pencils create a softer line than liquid liners, but you could also line eyes using eyeshadow powder and a small, pointed brush.

Mascara Choose from brown, brown/black or black for your everyday choice. One of these colours suits most people, and there is a fantastic variety of thickening, lengthening and curling formulas from which to choose.

Eyebrow pencil Useful for filling in sparse or overplucked brows, choose a pencil in no more than one shade darker than your natural brow colour. Alternatively, an eyeshadow powder can be brushed through your brows.

Lipstick Try to find a colour that is flattering even when you aren't wearing any other make-up. Experiment with different textures – matt, creamy, glossy and translucent – to find one that suits you.

Lip liner Choose a shade that matches your natural lip colour.

Lip gloss Tinted, clear and shimmery glosses are all available and can be used on their own or slicked on top of lipstick. Vaseline (petroleum jelly) provides many of the same advantages.

Shimmer Iridescent products are great for highlighting lips, lids, cheekbones and even shoulders. You can choose from cream, gel or powder formulas.

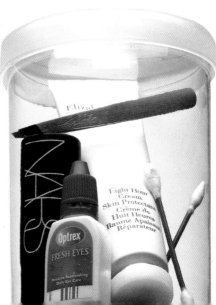

holiday and seasonal beauty

Whether the days are getting shorter and colder or you're jetting off to equatorial beaches, inevitably everything – your lifestyle, the food you eat, your exercise regime and your mood –will alter when the climate changes. During these times of transition it is important to keep the way in which you look after yourself in tune with your environment. Notice the effect changing climates and seasons have on your skin, hair and your whole being and adapt your beauty-care regime.

SUMMER/SPRING
- Exfoliate away dead, dry skin cells.
- Check that your moisturizer isn't too heavy, and choose one with an SPF of 15 or more.
- Consider switching to an oil-free moisturizer if you have skin that is prone to clogged pores in hot weather.

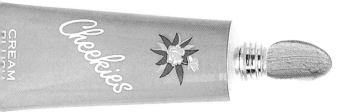

- Edit your make-up colours. Soft, feminine tones such as pinks and peachy hues are ideal for spring, whereas bright nail varnish and lip colours look great in the height of summer.
- Make-up should be minimal to allow skin to breathe – if you can't give it up completely, switch from a foundation to a tinted moisturizer.
- Now that your feet will be exposed, be sure to have – or give yourself – regular pedicures, and keep up with your manicures too.
- Start wearing a lighter fragrance – floral or citrus scents are best for the warmer months.
- Invest in a new hairstyle or colour (hair should be trimmed every eight weeks).
- Apply deep-conditioning hair treatments regularly to counteract the effects of exposure to sun, seawater and chlorine.

AUTUMN/WINTER

- This is the time to revert to 'real' make-up, so stock up on concealer, foundation and other necessities (see page 30–31).
- Check out the new season's colours and have fun experimenting with different looks to carry you through the winter months.
- Skin tends to become drier in the winter – so moisturize everywhere! Wear cotton gloves and socks to bed after lavishing a rich moisturizer all over your hands and feet to keep them soft.
- Check that your foundation is not too dark for your winter skin tone.
- Highlight your hair or try a rich new colour to lift drab winter days.

HOLIDAY TIME

Long-haul flights To prevent skin from dehydrating on long-haul flights, apply moisturizer frequently and drink plenty of water. Prevent static hair with a good grooming product.

Pack small Try to buy sample-size products for travelling or decant some of your own products into smaller plastic containers and bottles.

Sun protection Shielding your skin from the sun is important at all times so take good quality sun-protection (SPF 15 or over) products formulated for your face, body and lips.

Adventure breaks Think light and small. Take cleanser, a moisturizer, protective lip balm, sun protection, a decent hand cream and maybe mascara. Given that you are going to be outdoors, now is the time to forget the make-up bag and intensive skincare regime.

Beach holidays These are not meant to be high-maintenance experiences, so just pack the basics. Waterproof mascara is useful, but don't forget a deep-moisturizing hair mask if your locks have been overexposed to sun and saltwater.

City breaks Where you're going and the purpose will determine what you need to take. Pack your basic skincare products and try to choose multipurpose or compact items. Take your basic daytime make-up colours and deepen them for the evening.

Ski holidays Pack a moisturizer and lip block with an SPF of at least 25–30; skiing is extremely drying and you will be exposed to winds, intense UV rays and extremes of temperature. Keep make-up subtle on the slopes as it can look garish under such bright light.

Whoever described hair as our 'crowning glory' got it right. When your hair looks fabulous, you feel fabulous. Thinking back to your last bad hair day or disastrous cut is reminder enough of how important it is to be happy with your hair. And while a healthy diet, plenty of exercise and low stress levels all help build strong, healthy hair from the inside, what you apply externally is just as vital.

The latest products are designed to cope with specific needs, so if you really want to turn dull, unmanageable hair into sleek, glossy tresses, you simply have to buy the right products for your hair type. In the words of renowned trichologist, Philip Kingsley, 'good labelling should describe exactly what the product does and what hair type it's for – so be sure to check exactly what you're buying.' Kingsley strongly believes that a combination of regular cuts, good haircare and correct product usage will remedy most hair problems, including split ends and dandruff.

There are three basic hair types: fine, medium and thick. Fine hair, for example, usually needs volumizing products to add extra lift. On the other hand, thicker hair – along with hair that is coloured or damaged – tends to be drier and more porous; therefore, you need to use richer, more moisturizing formulations. It is also important to bear in mind any other difficulties you may have with your hair, such as oily roots or a flaky scalp.

Shampoos are basically designed to remove dirt, excess oil and dead skin cells from the scalp and hair. Contrary to popular belief, one wash is usually enough, unless you have a lot of product build-up. Regular use of conditioner will make hair softer, shinier and easier to comb through, plus protect it from heat and styling damage. Generally, the longer you leave a conditioner on, the more chance it has to attach itself to the cuticle and the better the results. Deep-conditioning treatments are a great once-a-week treat for parched hair. There are products available to protect hair and keep it in top condition, too.

Thermal styling lotions are applied to damp hair and work by forming a protective layer against heat damage from styling appliances. Similarly, many styling sprays and conditioners now contain UV filters to prevent colour fade or dryness.

Styling products (used correctly) are the perfect way to enhance your hairstyle, giving it extra hold and a glossy finish. Mousses work better on thicker hair, while lotions are ideal for finer locks, as they can be applied to the roots to give lift. Gels give texture to shorter styles and keep hair slicked down. Serums and shine products eliminate frizz, tame unruly hair and can add a supersleek finish to straight locks. Wax is best for giving definition to thicker hair, but it is too heavy for fine hair. Finally, a light mist of hairspray gives hold to any style or hair type. If you choose your hair products with the same care you would a face cream, you'll be rewarded with shiny, lustrous locks that are easier to manage.

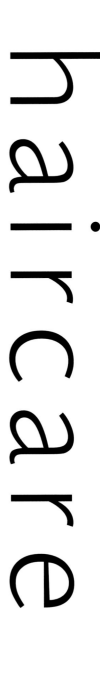

SHAMPOOS

◼ ALTERNA WEEKLY CLARIFYING SHAMPOO
Best shampoo for weekly use
£12.75 for 300ml
Great for thick or oily hair, this gentle shampoo detoxifies, removing all build-up
of pollution, smoke and residue from styling products, without stripping hair of its
natural oils. A base of plant ingredients helps to restore natural shine and retain
colour, while UV filters help protect hair from the sun.

◼ AUSSIE MEGA SHAMPOO
Best shampoo for daily use
£3.99 for 300ml
A superb everyday cleanser, this contains active ingredients such as blue gum
leaves and Australian mint balm. Scented with notes of peach, pineapple and
apple, it is a brilliant formula for shiny tresses, plus its lightweight formula will leave
hair full of natural body and bounce.

◼ AUSSIE SMOOTH MATE SHAMPOO
Best shampoo for flyaway hair
£3.99 for 300ml
The perfect solution to taming flyaway hair, this shampoo boasts the inclusion
of Australian blue gum leaves and stringy bark gum, which help control static and
smooth down excitable hair. Great for those damp days when hair is prone to frizz.

◼ AVEDA BLACK MALVA SHAMPOO
Best shampoo for dark shades
£7 for 250ml
Ideal for dark hair, this plant-based shampoo enriches hair colour while
discouraging the appearance of brassy or red tones in deeper shades. The key
ingredient in this product is black malva, a flowering herb known for its fantastic
moisturizing properties. After use, hair is left soft, manageable and glossy. It is
mild enough to use every day.

TIPS

- Good nutrition is mandatory for healthy, shiny hair. Make sure you eat
  a healthy, balanced diet that contains plenty of protein, carbohydrates,
  minerals, fat and vitamins.
- Ensure that you rinse all products thoroughly from your hair. Failure to do
  this will lead to limp, dull locks.
- Fine hair needs to be conditioned as much as other types, but only apply
  the product to the ends of the hair, and never to the scalp.
- Use a clarifying shampoo twice a month to reduce product build-up.

AVEDA SHAMPURE
Best shampoo for regular use
£8.50 for 250ml
A blend of 25 flower and plant essences – including coriander, eucalyptus, lavender and wheat – helps to make this light shampoo a celebrity favourite. Suitable for every hair type, it cleanses and conditions gently, leaving hair full of lustre and volume and smelling wonderfully fresh. It can be used daily, too.

BLACK LIKE ME REVITALIZING PROTEIN SHAMPOO
Best shampoo for Afro hair
£2.99 for 250ml
This is the one for thick or wiry Afro hair in need of a moisture fix. Packed with conditioning ingredients such as panthenol and silk amino acids, it achieves the perfect balance of cleansing hair without stripping it of its natural oils. Hair is left smooth and more manageable.

CHARLES WORTHINGTON DREAM HAIR UNBELIEVABLY CLEAN DETOX SHAMPOO
Best clarifying shampoo
£5.95 for 250ml
This fabulous product sweeps away dirt and styling overload without stripping your hair of its natural oils. It also has the added benefit of vitamin H, which replenishes both scalp and hair, leaving it shiny, bouncy and re-energized.

DANIEL FIELD SPRING WATER SHAMPOO
Best mild shampoo
£4.65 for 250ml
If your hair is suffering from product overkill, this mild shampoo will help restore its va va voom. Using it every day won't strip your hair and scalp of essential, natural oils, as some frequent-use shampoos do. Instead, hair is left clean and lightly conditioned.

DERMALOGICA SHINE THERAPY SHAMPOO
Best shampoo for brilliant shine
£18.60 for 237ml
This unique shampoo contains alphahydroxy citric acid – an ingredient usually found in skincare – which exfoliates and revitalizes both hair and scalp. Highlights are enhanced and the hair is endowed with bags of shine. It is best used once a week for a thorough cleanse.

DOVE 2 IN 1 MILK SHAMPOO
Best two-in-one shampoo
£2.59 for 250ml
Quite apart from being attractively priced, this is the ultimate buy when you're on the run and need a quick fix for supershiny locks. Like all Dove products, one

quarter of its contents comprises moisturizing milk to hydrate hair exceptionally, without weighing it down or leaving behind a dulling residue – a characteristic weakness among two-in-one shampoos.

FISH BIGFISH AMPLIFYING SHAMPOO
Best volumizing shampoo
£3.99 for 250ml
Deliciously fragranced with a blend of tropical coconut and grapefruit, this creamy shampoo deeply cleanses and nourishes and is excellent at creating body. Best volumizing results are achieved if hair is blow-dried after washing. Ideal for use on fine or limp hair that's in need of extra oomph.

JO HANSFORD PERFECT COLOUR SHAMPOO
Best shampoo for moisturizing coloured hair
£3.99 for 250ml
A mild shampoo designed to cleanse normal, colour-treated or highlighted hair gently. The formula contains UV filters to protect against sun damage and it can be used regularly. It also helps to reduce static by smoothing down the hair cuticle, leaving hair soft and full of shine.

JOHN FRIEDA SHEER BLONDE VOLUME ENHANCING SHAMPOO WITH HIGHLIGHT ACTIVATORS
Best shampoo for fine, blonde hair
£4.25 for 300ml
The first shampoo created specifically to add volume to natural, highlighted or colour-treated blonde hair, while enhancing its colour. It's packed with white grape juice, camomile, honey and wheatgerm extracts, which help rid hair of build-up and keep colour bright. Available in two formulations, one for platinum blondes and one for warmer, caramel shades.

JURLIQUE LAVENDER SHAMPOO
Best organic shampoo
£15.50 for 250ml
Free from chemicals, artificial preservatives, colourings and fragrances, Jurlique products are 100 per cent pure, natural and biodegradable. Rich in organic lavender and oils such as macadamia and jojoba, this shampoo is ideal for normal hair. Its highly concentrated formula means you need only use a tiny amount for beautiful, silky hair with a healthy shine.

KERASTASE NUTRITIVE SATIN BATH
Best shampoo for dry hair
£8.25 for 250ml
The ultimate turnaround treatment for parched hair, this extremely rich formula leaves even the driest hair silky and clean. It is designed to cleanse and moisturize hair deeply, without weighing it down or leaving it feeling heavy.

KERASTASE SOLEIL BAIN APRES-SOLEIL
Best shampoo for sun-exposed hair
£8 for 250ml

This concentrated shampoo is a rehydrating hair bath, designed to counteract the drying effects of sun, sea and chlorine. It is available in two formulations: one for coloured hair and one for hair that has not been treated. Both contain UV filters and pro-vitamin B5 to protect and restore lost moisture.

KLORANE OAT EXTRACT DRY SHAMPOO
Best dry shampoo
£5.45 for 200ml

If hectic schedules mean that you're always on the go, dry shampoo can be a life-saver and this is simply the best. It cleans without water, removing excess oil, dirt and dust in just a few minutes. Simply spray into your scalp and hair, then brush out. Hair is left feeling light and clean.

L'ANZA BE LONG CLEANSE SHAMPOO
Best shampoo if you're trying to grow your hair
£8.45 for 350ml

The perfect product for long hair, this gentle, conditioning shampoo stimulates hair growth, as well as helping to strengthen and protect existing hair. Its meadow foam seed oil and other natural ingredients work to leave hair shiny and tangle-free. Use every day if you are growing your hair.

L'OREAL PROFESSIONNEL SERIE EXPERT VITAMINO COLOUR SHAMPOO
Best shampoo for preventing colour fade
£5.75 for 250ml

This formula helps to stop colour fade and leaves hair gloriously glossy. It contains vitamins to condition damaged hair, and UV filters to protect your hair colour from the sun, helping to prolong its brilliance. It leaves hair smelling fresh and light, too.

MOLTON BROWN COOL MENTHA HAIR AND BODY SPORT WASH
Best shampoo for swimmers
£11 for 300ml

This tingly-fresh, all-in-one showering gel removes chlorine from your hair and body, while moisturizing all over. Containing menthol and refreshing citrus and spearmint oils, it stimulates and revives aching muscles after a swim. Ideal to take to the gym, as it will save you carrying two products.

MOP BASIL MINT SHAMPOO
Best deep-cleansing shampoo
£8.50 for 300ml

A gentle shampoo containing extracts of organic peppermint, basil, sage and rosemary that will really clean, clearing away all the dirt, pollution and oil that can build up in hair today, however careful we are, just because of the unseen air pollution that surrounds us. This shampoo will leave normal or oily hair lively, full of bounce and smelling wonderfully fresh. Suitable to use every day.

NEXXUS Y-SERUM SHAMPOO FOR YOUNGER LOOKING HAIR
Best shampoo for mature hair
£9.90 for 150ml

This anti-ageing shampoo contains extracts of green tea, shiitake mushrooms and other antioxidants, which help reduce the effects of ageing. Great for cleansing and revitalizing mature hair that has become dull or coarse with age. Use twice a week for healthier, more youthful-looking hair.

NICKY CLARKE COLOUR THERAPY TAKE IT AS RED SHAMPOO
Best shampoo for red hair
£4.99 for 250ml

This shampoo contains henna to add depth and shine to warm gold and red hair shades. It's bursting with natural ingredients including geranium, vanilla and coconut that help to leave hair silky-soft and smelling divine. All redheads should make this an essential feature of their bathroom.

ORIGINS THE LAST STRAW CONDITIONING SHAMPOO
Best shampoo for not needing conditioner
£12.50 for 200ml

Ideal for hair that has suffered abuse, whether that be from over-exposure to the sun, excessive colouring or the over use of heated hair appliances. Its luxurious cream base doesn't strip hair, infusing it instead with masses of moisture. And then extracts of vitamin E, wheat protein and apricot work to transform strawlike hair into shimmering strands. It leaves hair so soft that you won't need to use a conditioner afterwards.

OVER THE TOP SOUFFLE SHAMPOO
Best shampoo for brittle hair
£6.50 for 250ml

Another celebrity favourite, this shampoo contains a feast of nutrients such as sweet almond oil and aloe vera. It works up into a rich, creamy lather to cleanse hair gently, while adding moisture and body to every strand. Perfect for daily use on damaged hair that's sending out an SOS.

PANTENE PRO-V SHEER VOLUME SHAMPOO
Best budget volumizing shampoo
£1.99 for 200ml

Proven to increase lift by up to 80 per cent, this formula works instantly, building volume right from the roots. Enriched with pro-vitamin B5, which penetrates the hair shaft, it provides nourishment, adding texture and bounce. It's fabulous for fine hair, as it doesn't leave it feeling heavy.

PAUL MITCHELL TEA TREE SPECIAL SHAMPOO
Best shampoo for oily hair
£7.95 for 250ml

An invigorating product, this rids hair of everyday impurities. Moisturizing ingredients such as aloe vera, jojoba and henna are combined with Australian tea tree oil to leave even the lankest locks glossy and bouncy. The tingling sensation it creates on the scalp makes for a refreshing morning wake-up for hair.

PHILIP B ANTI-FLAKE SHAMPOO
Best shampoo for itchy scalps
£26.50 for 240ml

The ultimate rescue remedy for scalp-problem sufferers, this shampoo not only medicates, it also moisturizes and cleanses. A scalp-soothing blend of aloe vera, tea tree oil, juniper and camomile, it eases psoriasis and dandruff, providing long-lasting relief from flaking and itching.

PURE HAIR PATCHOULI BALANCING PURE SHAMPOO
Best shampoo for combination hair
£8.40 for 250ml

This shampoo is the answer if you have dry ends but greasy roots. A real hit with celebrities, it contains clove, patchouli and eight other essential oils, blended to deep-cleanse the scalp, while adding much-needed moisture to the hair tips.

REDKEN COLOUR EXTEND SHAMPOO
Best shampoo for preventing colour fade
£7.50 for 300ml

If you find your hair colour dulls quickly after the treatment, this is the perfect shampoo for you, as it helps guard against colour fade between salon visits. It's packed with proteins to strengthen hair, plus antioxidants and UV filters, which seal in colour, ensure a healthy shine and shield from the sun.

SPACE NK SOOTHING SHAMPOO
Best shampoo for sensitive scalps
£13.50 for 200ml

Designed to soothe allergy-prone and sensitive scalps, this shampoo cleanses gently, leaving hair shiny and manageable. The main active ingredients are aloe vera and oat extract – both know for their impressive skin-comforting properties.

TERAX BAMBINI SHAMPOO
Best baby shampoo
£6.95 for 250ml

Specially formulated to be ultra-gentle, making it a hit with babies – not to mention those delicate souls who need a little extra pampering. It cleanses gently, without stinging or bringing tears to the eyes, but still manages to achieve a thorough cleanse and leaves hair 'baby' soft and fresh-smelling.

TREVOR SORBIE PROFESSIONAL LONG HAIR RANGE – SHAMPOO FOR STRAIGHT HAIR
Best shampoo for long, straight hair
£4.99 for 300ml
Specifically formulated for long, straight hair, this shampoo contains a sunscreen, vitamin E and moisturizing agents that cleanse as well as protect, so hair is left knot-free and super-shiny. It is scented with notes of gardenia, lily and freesia for sweet-smelling locks.

CONDITIONERS

ALTERNA AGE-FREE PROTECTANT CONDITIONER
Best conditioner for mature hair
£19 for 500ml
Infused with caviar, which helps to increase hair's elasticity and strength, this rich conditioner rebalances moisture levels, protecting hair from the drying effects of ageing and the environment. Here is a great everyday conditioner to help restore youth to older hair.

ALTERNA ENZYMETHERAPY HEMP SEED ANTI-DANDRUFF CONDITIONER
Best conditioner for dandruff
£16.75 for 300ml
Containing organic extracts and willow bark, this deep-penetrating conditioner soothes an irritated scalp and prevents flaking to help control dandruff. Moisture-rich hemp seed oil adds shine and strength and prevents hair becoming frizzy. It's light enough for everyday use.

AUSSIE 3 MINUTE MIRACLE RECONSTRUCTOR
Best overall conditioner
£5.29 for 250ml
Apparently, more than 45 million bottles of this fabulous conditioner are sold worldwide each year. It's gentle enough for everyday use, whatever your hair type. Australian balm mint smoothes the hair's rough cuticles and penetrates deep within the shaft to reconstruct hair inside and out, as well as adding shine.

AVEDA BLUE MALVA CONDITIONER
Best conditioner for grey hair
£16 for 250ml
A great product that adds silvery brightness to grey hair, it also neutralizes any brassiness. With a base of natural plant ingredients, this almond-scented conditioner also helps seal the cuticles, giving hair dazzling shine. There are several different formulations, depending on your hair colour, including Camomile for blondes and Madder Root for brunettes.

BIOELEMENTS UNWIND DETANGLER
Best conditioner for frequent use
£23 for 150ml

This detangler and conditioner is full of natural ingredients such as shea butter and essential oils – orange, lavender, neroli, tangerine, petitgrain, grapefruit, rosemary and jojoba – which combine to moisturize and nourish both hair and scalp. It's designed to untangle knots and add shine without weighing down hair.

BUMBLE AND BUMBLE SEAWEED CONDITIONER
Best lightweight conditioner
£9.50 for 250ml

A favourite used devotedly by many catwalk models, this non-greasy, hydrating conditioner won't weigh down even the finest hair. Seaweed extract helps to detangle hair, leaving it easier to manage and shining with health.

CITRE SHINE SMOOTH OUT CONDITIONER
Best conditioner for creating shine
£3.49 for 300ml

This all-time favourite shine conditioner helps seal the hair cuticles, smoothing each strand as it goes and imparting incredible shine. Thanks to the light moisturizing properties of the citrus extracts and minerals, hair is left frizz-free, but doesn't feel heavy or weighed down.

DR HAUSCHKA HERBAL CONDITIONER
Best organic conditioner
£11 for 150ml

The organic herbal extracts in this conditioner work to balance the scalp's pH level and soften the hair, leaving it full of volume and revitalized. It is especially beneficial for a flaky scalp or dry, brittle hair.

IMAN NOURISHING CONDITIONING BALM
Best conditioner for Afro hair
£5.50 for 200ml

Light, creamy and detangling, this conditioner is specially designed to nourish Afro hair. The key ingredient is phytokeratin, a blend of botanical amino acids closely resembling proteins found naturally in hair. It helps to redress moisture balance, restoring shine and leaving hair smooth and supple.

JF LAZARTIGUE VITA-CREAM WITH MILK PROTEINS
Best conditioner for dry hair
£24 for 200ml

Both restorative and nourishing, this conditioner comes in two formulations, one for fine hair and one for normal hair. Apply, after washing, to towel-dried hair, focusing on the most damaged areas. Massage in and comb through, and then leave to work for up to ten minutes before rinsing.

JOHN FRIEDA SHEER BLONDE VOLUME PRESERVING DETANGLER
Best conditioner for adding volume to blonde hair
£4.25 for £250ml

Blonde hair tends to be finer than other hair colours, which makes it more delicate and prone to snagging and snarling. As it is combed through, this ultra-light conditioner helps to protect fragile hair from tearing, while also making hair thicker and full of body, and brightening blonde tones.

JOICO K-PACK LEAVE-IN PROTECTANT
Best leave-in conditioner
£7.95 for 300ml

This conditioner creates sensational shine and nourishes all hair types but the kulhui nut and guava extract it contains is especially good for reconstructing dry, tired hair without leaving it lank and greasy. Its unique foaming formula helps to seal moisture into hair, protecting it from heat damage caused by frequent styling.

KERASTASE DERMO CALM CONDITIONER
Best conditioner for sensitive scalps
£8.25 for 250ml

Most conditioners should be used only on the hair lengths and ends, but this product calms and soothes irritable scalps, too, so it can be used all over. A small amount should be applied to the roots then massaged through the rest of the hair.

KERASTASE MASQUINTENSE
Best intensive conditioner
£11 for 150ml

This conditioner is available in two formulations, one for fine hair and one for thick hair. Both add body and shine by smoothing the cuticles, leaving hair glossy and tangle-free. If your hair is very badly damaged, you can leave it on for longer than the recommended ten minutes.

KERASTASE RESISTANCE CIMENT ANTI-WEAR
Best conditioner for chemically treated hair
£9.50 for 200ml

Whether your hair is damaged through too much blow-drying, an abrasive shampoo or an overdose of colour treatments, this intense conditioner is a marvellous restorative. Use it every couple of months as a serious pick-me-up.

KIEHL'S EXTRA STRENGTH CONDITIONING RINSE
Best conditioner for very damaged hair
£17 for 200ml

This thick conditioner, enriched with panthenol, keratin and coconut, will detangle and give renewed strength, body and shine to stressed strands. Apply generously to clean, damp hair, concentrating on the ends, then leave for five minutes and rinse. With regular use it will leave hair more robust and less prone to breakage.

KLORANE MACASSAR NOURISHING CREAM
Best conditioner for very dehydrated hair
£5.95 for 200ml

If your hair is suffering from extreme dryness due to overindulgence in colour, perms or straightening treatments, this is the conditioner for you. Containing extract of macassar, a plant oil that has been used as a natural hair softener for thousands of years, the conditioner nourishes and rehydrates even the most devitalized hair, restoring softness and shine. Use it every day until the condition of your hair improves.

KMS AMP VOLUME RECONSTRUCTOR
Best thickening conditioner
£7.95 for 250ml

This deep-penetrating body builder is perfect for thinning hair. It contains amino acids and wheat proteins, which penetrate the hair shaft to add thickness to individual strands, so your hair is left looking fuller. Hair strength is improved too, which reduces the risk of breakage.

L'OREAL ELVIVE SMOOTH-INTENSE CONDITIONER WITH NUTRILEUM
Best conditioner for unmanageable hair
£2.49 for 200ml

Penetrating deep into the hair follicles, this anti-frizz conditioner also smoothes and calms dry, damaged ends, giving a lasting shine from root to scalp. It contains nutrileum, a derivative of silicone that can help to strengthen hair, so it's great for dry, hard-to-control coarse hair, giving definition and softness to unruly locks. Used regularly, it will improve the manageability of your hair.

MATRIX BIOLAGE COLOUR CARE CONDITIONER
Best conditioner for preventing colour fade
£6.45 for 250ml

This nourishing conditioner locks in hair colour, stopping it from fading while intensifying shine at the same time. It contains extracts of nettle and sunflower seed oil, which work to moisturize hair, leaving it tangle-free and glossy. As a bonus, the conditioner boasts natural sun filters that help to shield hair from UV damage. It can be used every day on colour-treated hair.

MOP LEMONGRASS CONDITIONER
Best conditioner for fine hair
£8.95 for 300ml

This product is great for those who suffer from limp locks. It is a botanical conditioner containing extracts of lemongrass and camomile to promote shine and body and to keep excess oil under control, and honey and wheatgerm to nourish the hair naturally and to help to maintain elasticity. After treatment hair is left fresh and full of bounce, with no unwanted weight.

NEUTROGENA CLEAN REVIVING CONDITIONER
Best conditioner for oily hair
£2.99 for 300ml

An oil-free conditioner, this is the business for hair that tends to be greasy. It is intense enough to remove tangles and leave ends smooth, while the light formula contains panthenol for added strength and shine, without leaving behind any dulling build-up. Hair is fragranced with a fresh, clean scent, and given gratifying fullness and sheen.

PANTENE PRO-V COMPLETE CARE CONDITIONER
Best budget conditioner
£1.99 for 200ml

Designed to combat the six signs of unhealthy hair – weakness, split ends, dryness, plus lack of shine, manageability and body – this conditioner is based on a pro-vitamin B formula that helps to protect and renourish. Only a tiny amount is needed to leave hair feeling silky and bouncing with health.

PAUL MITCHELL THE CONDITIONER
Best anti-static conditioner
£6.85 for 250ml

A light, daily conditioner for all hair types, this leave-in formula helps to nourish hair and protect it from the wear and tear of daily styling. Awaphui extract is absorbed into the hair, softening it, without leaving build up behind, and hair is left easy to comb through. The product also doubles as a soothing body moisturizer. A little goes a long way, so a thumbnail-sized blob is enough for most hair lengths.

PHILIP KINGSLEY BODY BUILDING CONDITIONER
Best conditioner for limp hair
£11.95 for 200ml

This prime product from renowned trichologist Philip Kingsley is the answer for limp, droopy hair. Its lightweight formula coats each individual strand of hair, sealing in moisture and adding much-needed body and shine – without the heaviness of some conditioners. As an added bonus, it helps to protect hair from blow-drying.

PHILOSOPHY THE BIG BLOW OFF
Best spray conditioner
£9.50 for 236.6ml

Hairdryer junkies should take good note of this one: an oil-free spray conditioner that will help to protect your hair from heat burn-out. Just spritz a small amount on to towel-dried, damp hair and comb it through. The formula contains pro-vitamin B5, which will strengthen hair and reduce damage, together with vegetable proteins, which will add body to fine hair. It can also be used as a handy standby to smooth down frizz during the day.

PHYTO SPECIFIC VITAL FORCE CREME BATH
Best conditioner for curly hair
£17.50 for 200ml
Formulated specifically for naturally curly or frizzy hair, this quality product contains plant extracts and wheat proteins to hydrate and protect hair. After just one application your curls will be easier to style and will look glossier and healthier.

PURE HAIR BASIL MINT DETANGLING ELIXIR
Best conditioner for detangling long hair
£8.40 for 250ml
An equalizing, light conditioner, this is infused with organic extracts of basil and essential oils such as peppermint and rosemary. Its lightweight formula means even the longest hair is left soft and knot-free.

SEBASTIAN TITANIUM PROTECTOR
Best protecting conditioner
£10.50 for 250ml
This conditioner forms an invisible coat of armour around each hair, protecting it from heated styling and the environment. It is suitable for all hair types and, remarkably, it is light enough to use every day.

TERAX ORIGINAL CREMA
Best for preventing split ends
£8.25 for 150ml
This conditioner – among Madonna's favourites – has wonderful softening properties and helps to restore the hair's normal pH level. It relieves dryness, split ends and static and will bring vitality back to even chemically treated hair.

TE TAO WARM HENNA RED NATURAL COLOUR PROTECT CONDITIONER
Best conditioner for red hair
£3.95 for 300ml
Combining the principles of Chinese herbal medicine with natural plant ingredients, this conditioner helps enhance and maintain the colour and warmth of red and auburn hair. It contains madder root and henna, two herbs known to boost colour intensity and promote shine.

TREVOR SORBIE MOISTURIZING AND DE-FRIZZING RICH CONDITIONER
Best basic conditioner for flyaway hair
£4.49 for 250ml
A rich conditioner, ideal for hair that knots and tangles easily, this targets and treats weakened areas, replenishing moisture and taming flyaway ends – and it's packed with antioxidants such as grapeseed extract, green tea and vitamin E, which help to protect hair against further damage. The result? Smooth, easy-to-manage hair.

TREATMENTS AND MASKS

ANDREW COLLINGE SALON SOLUTIONS 1 MINUTE WONDER
Best treatment for damaged hair
99p per 25ml sachet
Sun, heated styling appliances and colouring can all take their toll on hair, leaving it dry and brittle. This deep-penetrating treatment quickly restructures damaged hair. Formulated to lock in moisture, it leaves hair soft and supple and also contains protective multivitamins and UV filters. It makes a good weekly treat for parched hair in need of rescue.

BIOELEMENTS SCALP SPECIALIST
Best treatment for a healthy scalp
£22 for 118ml
This exhilarating pre-shampoo gel stimulates circulation to nourish hair roots and exfoliates follicle-clogging flakes, thus allowing hair to grow better and stronger, while soothing an itchy scalp in the process. Tingling menthol is the main ingredient of this product, which is simply massaged directly into the scalp for a minute before shampooing. Use once a week.

BLACK LIKE ME REVITALIZING TREATMENT
Best treatment for Afro hair
£5.98 for 250ml
This is a rich product, ideal for hair that has been chemically relaxed. Jojoba oil and keratin are absorbed deep into the hair shaft which leaves otherwise unruly locks shiny and much easier to manage. It is excellent for preventing mid-length hair breakages and split ends.

BORGHESE FANGO ACTIVE MUD FOR HAIR AND SCALP
Best treatment for lifeless hair
£33 for 500g
A mineral-enriched, volcanic-mud formulation that invigorates even the most devitalized hair, this also boasts essential oils of geranium, lavender and peppermint. It's deeply cleansing and moisturizing, and even adds volume and shine. Apply to dry hair and allow to work its magic for between five and ten minutes before rinsing, then shampoo and style as usual. Use the mud twice a month to rejuvenate scalp and tresses.

DANIEL GALVIN COLOUR SHINE BRIGHTENER
Best treatment for lifting faded colour
£4.99 for one application
'King of colour' Daniel Galvin calls this his 'miracle solution' for revitalizing hair colour and highlights. Just one application of this gentle product restores brightness, leaving your hair colour almost as glossy as the day it was done. It is a great way to keep hair looking fresh between salon visits.

DANIEL GALVIN PRE-COLOUR CLEANSER
Best colour-preparation treatment product
£3.99 for one application
Handy to use the day before you colour your hair, this product removes pollution
and styling build-up, creating a clean base for the colour to 'take' better. The mild
vitamin C formulation means hair isn't overstripped but remains soft and shiny.

E'SPA PINK HAIR AND SCALP MUD
Best scalp-soothing treatment
£26 for 200g
This intensive treatment revitalizes dry or chemically treated hair. It contains
mineral-rich red clay, plus watercress and apricot kernel oil, to help condition your
hair and scalp. It can also be left in dry or wet hair while sunbathing or swimming,
to protect against the damaging effects of UV light and chlorine.

FISH FOOD FISH CAKE NOURISHING CLAY HAIR MASK
Best treatment for hair dulled by residue and pollution build-up
£7.49 for 200ml
To cleanse and detoxify, white clay is the base for this megastrength restorative
mask. Filled with natural goodies such as avocado oil and peppermint, it's
guaranteed to leave hair looking and feeling gorgeous. Use once a fortnight to
give a hair a pampering home spa treat.

FRESH ILLIPE BUTTER DEEP CONDITIONER
Best all-round conditioning treatment
£19.50 for 150ml
This product should be used once a week as an intensive repair mask. Illipe butter
is rich in natural fatty acids, and has extraordinary moisturizing properties to
condition the scalp and transform frizz into smooth, citrus-scented glossy locks.

GARNIER FRUCTIS INTENSE COLOUR LAST MASK
Best treatment for coloured hair
£3.99 for 150ml
If your hair has been coloured or highlighted, this reasonably priced treatment
mask contains avocado and apricot oils, which help to lock in colour and make
it last longer, while moisturizing hair deeply. It is designed to work in two to three
minutes and gives remarkable results.

**HEALTHY SEXY HAIR CONCEPTS SOY FUEL POWER
CONDITIONING BOOSTER**
Best booster treatment
£14.35 for 30ml
Just add a few drops of this boosting oil to your usual conditioner to create a
superconditioner. It's packed with soya protein and moisturizing botanicals to
make hair stronger and bouncier. Use twice a week to guarantee high-octane hair.

HEALTHY SEXY HAIR SOY POTION MIRACULOUS LEAVE-IN TREATMENT
Best for very dry hair
£12.35 for 150ml

This gel-based, leave-in treatment contains soy to revive ultra-dry hair. Despite being light, it's able to drench hair powerfully with moisture, using a mixture of jojoba, macadamia and evening primrose oils. Scented with mango and ginger, this is the ultimate turnaround treatment for really dry hair.

JOHN FRIEDA BEACH BLONDE KELP HELP DEEP CONDITIONING MASQUE
Best treatment for sun-frazzled blonde hair
£4.95 for 100ml

This is a beach-time essential that should be in every blonde's suitcase. Containing a combination of protein-rich algae, aloe vera and vitamin E, this treatment infuses sun-damaged hair with moisture and suppleness. Added UV protectors help guard against further drying.

KERASTASE FORCINTENSE DOSAGE VITA-CIMENT
Best treatment for severely weakened hair
£17.50 for 5x15ml

If your hair is very damaged and suffering from overprocessing, this is the product to restore it to good health. The revitalizing Vita-Ciment Complex it contains is absorbed into the hair, strengthening it from the inside out. After only five applications, breakage and splitting is reduced, leaving you with healthy, shiny hair.

L'ANZA BE LONG STRENGTHEN
Best treatment for strengthening long hair
£9.20 for 150ml

This product is designed to increase the potential length that hair can grow to, by providing strength and shine for the older part of the hair that is lower down the shaft – and may be two- or three-years-old. It should be used after shampooing, two to three times a week.

TIPS

- Treat your hair to a deep, intensive conditioner or mask once a week in order to keep it in prime condition.
- Hot oils are a great way to put condition back into frayed, damaged hair.
- Mix an egg yolk and an overripe avocado for an at-home conditioning treatment for dry, damaged hair. Leave on for 30 minutes before rinsing.
- Use a good quality hair protector when in the sun, salt water or chlorine.
- Try conditioning your hair while you lie in the sun. Wet your hair, smooth on the conditioner and relax for 20 minutes, letting the sun do all the work.

L'OREAL PROFESSIONNEL SERIE EXPERT INTENSE REPAIR NUTRITION MASK
Best treatment for flyaway hair
£7.25 for 150ml

Deeply nourishing to condition dry lengths and ends, this mask contains amino acids and vitamin B6 to help to detangle and smooth hair, imbuing it with a beautiful sheen. While it is rich enough to revitalize dry and damaged locks, it doesn't weigh hair down. Don't be infuriated by fine flyaway hair, give it some serious pampering instead: this mask could become a great weekly treat.

OVER THE TOP INSTANT FEEDBACK INTENSE PENETRATING TREATMENT
Best treatment for tired, lacklustre hair
£8.50 for 125ml

One of the most effective deep conditioners around, this one is just perfect for hair that has become dull and lifeless. A combination of sweet almond oil, pro-vitamin B5 and vitamin E nourishes and strengthens the hair. But best of all, it takes only three minutes to work, making it marvellous when you're in a hurry but want instantly better-looking hair.

PHILIP B REJUVENATING OIL
Best treatment for split ends
£22.50 for 60ml

This nourishing oil, containing a blend of carrier oils and sensual essential oils including lavender, geranium and ylang-ylang, closely replicates the scalp's own natural oils. Really working in the oil thoroughly from the roots through to the ends encourages the treatment to penetrate deep into the hair shaft, reviving tired locks and increasing elasticity.

PHILIP KINGSLEY ELASTICIZER
Best treatment for lank hair
£16.50 for 150ml

This highly concentrated treatment improves the suppleness and flexibility of your hair, providing extra shine and manageability. For best results, apply to damp hair, wrap hair in a hot, moist towel for about five minutes, then rinse and shampoo as normal. Use once a week.

PHYTO PHYTOCITRUS ESSENTIAL NUTRITION HAIR MASK
Best treatment for chemically treated hair
£15 for 200ml

This botanical, deep-nourishing mask revitalizes hair that has been dried out by frequent colouring and perming. It combines extracts of grapefruit and shea butter, which not only restore the hair's natural elasticity, but help to minimize colour fade as well. The formula also contains UV filters to protect hair from unavoidable environmental damage, too.

PHYTO PHYTOCYANE THINNING HAIR TREATMENT
Best treatment for thinning hair
£27 for 12 ampoules

This is an effective answer to the first stage of hair loss in women, which can be triggered by stress, poor diet or hormonal imbalances. Its cocktail of amino acids, vitamins and ginkgo biloba boosts circulation and helps to stimulate hair regrowth. Use daily to prevent further hair loss.

REDKEN ALL SOFT HEAVY CREAM
Best treatment for wiry hair
£13.50 for 250ml

This superconditioning treatment provides an intensive moisture boost for coarse hair. The cream contains jojoba and avocado oil, which penetrates the hair shaft to soften and control frizz, making this an ideal treatment for damaged or naturally curly hair in need of improved condition and control.

SCHWARZKOPF BONACURE BI-PHASE TREATMENT
Best treatment for hair prone to breakage
£15.50 for 2x100ml

Apply this in two steps: the first treatment contains proteins to penetrate the hair and build strength within its fibres, the second has honey extract to smooth the hair's cuticles. Hair is left soft and with added protection from external damage, for up to five washes. Use whenever hair feels particularly dry.

UMBERTO GIANNINI URGENT REPAIR INTENSE MOISTURE MASK
Best treatment for stressed hair
£5.95 for 200ml

Used weekly, this deep-working wonder treatment will revitalize lacklustre locks; it penetrates the hair deeply to nourish and repair even the most worn and torn tresses. Work into the lengths and ends of hair, leave for ten minutes, and rinse.

WELLA ADVANCED VO5 HOT OIL
Best treatment for brittle hair
£2.99 for 3x15ml tubes

This trusted and well-priced classic reconstructs damaged hair in just one minute and reduces breakage by up to 60 per cent. It's designed to leave behind only as much moisture as hair needs, by targeting the most damaged areas. Whatever is not required simply washes away. Hair is left soft and silky for up to four washes. Always use before shampooing.

WELEDA ROSEMARY HAIR LOTION
Best natural treatment
£4.35 for 100ml

Among the ingredients of this therapeutic lotion, alongside extracts of sedum and horseradish, is rosemary, a herb that has been used for centuries for its stimulating

properties to cure dry hair and scalps, leaving hair ultra-shiny and easy to man
Regular use will improve the condition of permed and bleached hair particularly,
daily use will add body to hair, making it appear fuller and thicker.

WELLA VITALITY REPAIR AND CARE TREATMENT
Best treatment for lifeless hair
£1.25 for 25ml
A product with an attractive price, containing rich protein extracts to replenish
and strengthen the structure of your hair. A three-minute application will leave
hair repaired, intensively conditioned and protected against further damage.

STYLING PRODUCTS

AVEDA HANG STRAIGHT STRAIGHTENING LOTION
Best straightening product
£14 for 200ml
Excellent for achieving poker-straight hair, smoothing and taming flyaway
strands. It contains organic marshmallow root and flaxseed extract for hold,
plus natural silica to enhance shine and defy fuzziness. Wash hair, apply a small
amount of the lotion and style as normal.

BLACK AND WHITE HAIR WAX
Best product for Afro hair
£3.99 for 50ml
A cult classic that originates from Jamaica, revered there as the antidote for the
Caribbean bad hair day. Nowadays it's used all over the world by those with
unruly hair who love its versatility. This product can't be beaten when it comes to
smoothing and holding styles in place.

BUMBLE AND BUMBLE HAIR POWDER
Best product for texture and grip
£10.90 for 200g
A favourite of the session stylist, this innovative bestselling product is designed to
help create ultra-modern styles. Just spray a little of the fine powder into your hair
and you'll have lots of volume and a dry, matt appearance that helps to absorb the
light. It also gives hair fantastic grip, making it ideal for keeping 'up-dos' up.

CHARLES WORTHINGTON PERFECT REFLECTION PROTECT AND SHINE TEXTURIZING WAX FOR DARK SHADES
Best product for adding evening glamour to dark hair
£7.99 for 50ml
This clever product contains light reflectors and tiny particles of shimmer so hair
glistens in the light, while the wax defines and controls your hairstyle. One
fingertip-sized blob is enough for most hair lengths.

CHARLES WORTHINGTON RESULTS RELAX AND UNWIND BLOW-DRY STRAIGHTENING BALM
Best product for taming unruly hair
£3.95 for 200ml

Iron out rebellious waves and kinks with this straightening balm that coaxes even the frizziest hair into submission. Apply to damp hair before blow-drying, for a sleek, smooth style. It leaves hair with a high-shine finish and smelling heavenly, too.

CITRE SHINE WOUND UP CURLING MOUSSE
Best product for controlling curls
£3.99 for 250ml

Infused with shine-enhancing citrus extract, plus vitamins and minerals to help protect hair from the environment, this mousse will tame frizz and cultivate curls and natural-looking waves, imparting bounce, control and sheen.

CLAIROL HERBAL ESSENCES VOLUMIZING ROOT LIFTER
Best budget volumizer
£2.99 for 175ml

A great find for hair that requires added body and vitality. Apply directly to the roots after washing to add thickness and shine to limp hair. Its unique blend of chrysanthemum, orange blossom and caraway extract leaves hair smelling fresh and sweetly fragranced as well as looking big and beautiful.

CLINIQUE LIGHT CONTROL GEL
Best control product for longer styles
£10 for 150ml

This gel is great for taming hair that is at the in-between stage of growing out, but offers long-wearing, flexible hold suitable for all hair types. It contains polymers to smooth the hair shaft and reduce frizz, and panthenol to add sleekness and shine. It has a soft, non-sticky texture and it's alcohol-free, so it won't dry out your hair.

CLINIQUE STRONG HOLD GEL
Best control product for short styles
£10 for 150ml

Allergy-tested and 100 per cent fragrance-free, this gel can be applied to either wet or dry hair, before or after styling. It gives lasting, strong hold to shorter styles. Formulated with moisturizers that stop hair feeling or looking dry, it makes hair stay put in damp, humid weather.

FRESH SHAPING FOAM
Best product for bounciness
£16 for 150ml

This product takes the body-building benefits of panthenol and adds soybean extract and wheat protein as volumizers, to offer soft hold with plenty of oomph, and bergamot extract, to stimulate the scalp and leave hair smelling gorgeous.

FUDGE HAIR PUTTY
Best product for height
£2.95 for 30ml
This unique moulding clay gives styles height and lift, while keeping hair in good condition and with a healthy sheen – and it's almond-scented so hair smells as great as it looks. Work a small amount through the roots, down to the mid-lengths of damp hair, to add impressive lift.

GARNIER FRUCTIS SPRITZ GEL
Best product for a lasting hold
£3.99 for 300ml
Slightly fragranced, this gel is the perfect product for any style that requires some serious hold. Its clear formula turns to liquid when sprayed on hair, giving every strand extra volume, contrast and hold – without stickiness or stiffness.

HEALTHY SEXY HAIR CONCEPTS SHATTER
Best for short, sassy styles
£9.45 for 125ml
If you're bored of sleek locks and long for a more tousled look, this is the product for you. A few squirts of its pump spray can instantly turn short, cropped styles into chic, fragmented locks. As well as offering firm hold, it also separates the hair. Apply to dry hair, pulling out a few pieces to create a shattered style.

JOHN FRIEDA BEACH BLONDE GOLD RUSH SHIMMER GEL
Best product for adding evening glamour to blonde hair
£5.50 for 100ml
Perfect for a special night out, this is a soft-control gel, infused with little pieces of gold to give hair ultimate sparkle. You can paint it on as instant highlights or use it to brighten up root regrowth if you've not had time to get to the salon.

KERASTASE NUTRITIVE OLEO-RELAX
Best for rebellious hair
£12.50 for 125ml
You can discipline the wildest locks with this controlling serum. It combines shorea oil and palm tree oil to soften, smooth and ensure frizz-free, shiny hair. Added UV filters help to protect hair from the frazzling effects of the sun, so you should slip this into your suitcase on sunny holidays abroad.

KIEHL'S CREME WITH SILK GROOM
Best overall styling product
£17.50 for 100ml
A favourite of hairdressers since its creation in the 1970s, this cream delivers terrific texture, suppleness and shine. It contains silk amino acids and easily absorbed oils to control and define most hairstyles. Rub into palms and apply to wet hair before styling, or use sparingly on dry hair for a sleeker-than-sleek finish.

L'OREAL PROFESSIONNEL TECNI.ART A.HEAD ZAPP MODELLING STICK
Best product for spiky styles
£9.99 for 75ml
This must-have product for cropped hair comes in a handy stick, which allows you to apply it directly into hair, for more precise styling. Plus it gives sensational shine and a light, non-greasy hold. Perfect for defining spiky textures.

MICHAELJOHN SALONSPA ROOT LIFT THICKENING SPRAY
Best product for adding root lift
£4.99 for 250ml
Aromatherapy essences, including those of lavender, camomile and juniper berry, work to revive tired hair and add fullness and shine. Just spray onto the roots and each strand acquires lift and bounce. It also contains vitamin E and sunscreens to protect hair from damaging UV light.

MULTIPLICITY TOUSLE CREAM 'N' GEL
Best non-sticky product
£6.95 for 50g
A dual-purpose styler that manages to combine a cream that smoothes hair, leaving it glossy, with a moderate-hold gel to give style and shape. This is the one when you want to create a messy, less structured style that doesn't feel tacky to touch.

NEXXUS EXXTRA GEL
Best product for 'wet-look' styles
£10.50 for 400ml
This spray gel is ideal for light hair sculpting. It contains a mixture of collagen, amino acids and elastins to add strength, elasticity and shine to hair, yet is free from dulling residues and drying alcohol so doesn't leave hair feeling brittle. Your best bet if you want to create a wet-look style.

PAUL MITCHELL STRAIGHT WORKS
Best product for defining curls
£7.25 for 100ml
A lightweight gel that transforms even the most unruly, unmanageable hair into dead-straight styles. It works by helping to reduce the wave of naturally curly hair, and creates a shiny, silky-smooth finish.

PHILIP B DEAD STRAIGHTENING BALM
Best product for hard-to-straighten hair
£16 for 192ml
Even die-hard curls go straight when treated with this product. It conjures shiny, bouncy hair using extracts of matricaria and horseradish and an acrylic polymer. Unlike some straightening lotions, this balm is non-greasy and water-soluble, so hair doesn't feel heavy or suffer from dulling product build-up.

PHYTO PHYTOVOLUME MAXIMIZING VOLUME SPRAY
Best product for adding volume to fine hair
£10 for 100ml

This is marvellous for volumizing fine, limp hair. It coats and reinforces hair to increase overall volume and add bounce and vitality. Containing nasturtium and beetroot extracts, it holds styles well and bestows a dazzling shine. For best results, apply it after washing and then blow-dry.

REDKEN SMART WAX
Best smoothing product
£8.50 for 50ml

For an extra-smooth finish, apply this heat-sensitive wax to just-washed hair, then blow-dry as normal. For a more 'mussed-up' look, simply switch your hairdryer to cold. A versatile product ideal for giving a polished look to most styles and suitable for all hair types, too.

REDKEN TRUE CALM LIGHT STYLER AND RESTYLER
Best product for light support
£10.50 for 250ml

This leave-in spray is formulated with camomile for its hydrating properties and a variety of natural oils that work to smooth and tame. Apply to towel-dried hair after shampooing, then style. It can be reapplied at any time during the day to refresh a style.

SEBASTIAN THREADS
Best product for fringes
£16.50 for 100ml

Give striking definition to fringes with this light-control hair cream. It can be used to separate individual strands for a 'piecey' look and lasts all day, without leaving your fringe feeling greasy or weighed down. Apply a tiny amount to dry hair.

SEBASTIAN XTAH DIRTY WORKS
Best dual-purpose product
£16.50 for 125ml

A great dual-purpose conditioner and styler in one. Simply massage in after shampooing, then wash out, for a conditioning treat. Alternatively, leave it in without rinsing for added moisture and manageability. It provides medium hold and is suitable for all hair types.

TIGI BEDHEAD SMALL TALK
Best volumizing product
£11 for 200ml

This non-sticky lotion puts the life back into your hair. It provides good control and plenty of definition to limp locks, and smells of delicious blueberry. Use on wet or dry hair for added height and lift.

TIGI BEDHEAD SMALL TALK THICKIFIER
Best product for layered hair
£11 for 42g
A three-in-one thickening, energizing and styling cream, not only does this add body to limp, lifeless hair, it also styles and separates. Just one fingertip-sized blob is enough to define the layers in longer hair.

TIGI CATFIGHT PLIABLE PUDDING
Best product for adding texture
£11 for 42g
This bright purple stickyness can be run through the mid-lengths of wet or dry hair to create a textured, sharp finish that is flexible but long-lasting. It also smoothes and conditions the hair cuticle as it styles, leaving the hair healthily shiny.

TONI AND GUY BOOST IT MOUSSE
Best for dry or coloured hair
£5.99 for 250ml
This mousse controls, holds and adds noticeable volume. It's ideal for use on damaged locks as its added moisturizers nourish hair while it holds a style. Concentrating on the roots, apply one golf-ball-sized blob before blow-drying.

TREVOR SORBIE CURL CREAM
Best product for defining curly hair
£4.99 for 150ml
A rich cream that conditions each strand to give a high-gloss, tangle-free, medium-hold finish to curly hair, making it bouncier, smoother and full of shine. Apply the cream generously to damp hair, and then, for tumbling curls, use your fingers to separate; for springy curls, scrunch up; and for spirals, twist small sections around your finger.

UMBERTO GIANNINI UPLIFTING THICKENING MOUSSE
Best product for holding fine, limp hair
£3.95 for 200ml
Light, and non-sticky, this mousse gives maximum hold to all styles and contains shine-enhancing ingredients, including wheat proteins and polymers that also help to thicken each hair. After shampooing, apply enough product to coat hair completely and comb through before styling.

URBAN THERAPY TWISTED SISTA CURL ACTIVATOR
Best curl-reviving product
£2.50 for 200ml
The remedy for drooping, tired curls, this product delivers volume, bounce and definition to naturally curly or permed hair. Squeeze a generous amount into your hands, then run through hair from roots to tips. A handy dressing-table essential for every curly girl.

WELLA HIGH HAIR OCEAN SPRITZ
Best product for the tousled look
£5.70 for 125ml
Designed to recreate that 'just stepped out of the sea' surf-chick look, this funky product deploys salt water as its magic ingredient. Just spray into damp hair, scrunch and allow to dry naturally or with a diffuser for tousled sex appeal. A good bargain, performing like a more expensive product, but at half the price.

SERUMS/SHINE PRODUCTS

ALTERNA HEMP SEED POLISHING GLOSS
Best for adding shine to frizzy hair
£12.75 for 70ml
Afro or wiry hair often needs extra help and a dollop of cult haircare company Alterna's gloss will separate and tame even the wildest hair. Its seaweed extracts will reduce static as the hemp seed oil increases hair's elasticity and shine.

AVEDA LIGHT ELEMENTS SMOOTHING FLUID
Best botanical shine product
£5.99 for 100ml
This styling liquid provides movement and restores a healthy sheen to your hair. Plant-based ingredients, such as organic jojoba, condition hair at the same time as adding natural body and shine, which explains why this product is popular with hairdressers around the world.

CITRE SHINE MIRACLE HAIR POLISHER
Best for dull hair
£4.95 for 30ml
This polishing product smoothes and seals the hair cuticles and contains citrus extract to impart brilliant shine to even the dullest locks. It also helps detangle and improve hair's manageability, for easier styling.

TIPS

- Use serums sparingly, because hair can get weighed down easily and become greasy.
- To straighten hair, apply a few drops of serum before blow-drying, slicking it into your palms and then running it over your hair to disperse evenly.
- Use styling products correctly: a styling cream should be applied before using a heating appliance; a mousse is designed to give volume and body, so apply it before blow-drying; thickening creams style and set the hair and are also applied to damp hair before styling; and serums help to control frizz or to define curls, apply these to wet or dry hair before or after styling.

CLINIQUE HAIR CARE HEALTHY SHINE SERUM
Best for weakened hair
£10 for 150ml
This serum softens and protects hair from the ravages of the seasons and air-conditioning, while helping to maximize shine. Its lightweight formula is also water-resistant so it will continue to keep hair smooth even if it gets wet.

CLYNOL HAIR SHINE SPRAY
Best spray-on shine
£4.90 for 150ml
This all-time favourite shine product has been specially formulated to give hair sheen and softness. Its light formula not only provides long-lasting shine and improves the appearance of dry, porous hair, but does so without causing build-up or making hair feel dirty. It can also be used to protect hair ends from blow-drying and environmental damage.

JO HANSFORD SEAL AND SHINE SERUM
Best for coloured hair
£5.99 for 50ml
A high shine, ultra-light serum, this is designed to defrizz colour-treated hair. Apply a few drops to damp hair and work through to help eliminate frizz and prevent colour fade.

JOICO K-PAC RECONSTRUCTOR PROTECT AND SHINE SERUM
Best for split ends
£11.99 for 50ml
This rich serum treats hair, protecting it from damage while adding shine. Its unique formula actually helps to repair damaged hair. Rub a little on the bottom of dry or wet hair to seal split ends.

MATRIX SLEEK LOOK WATER-FREE LOCKDOWN SPRAY
Best for heat-styled hair
£7.90 for 125ml
This supershiny formula is designed to lock in moisture and provide hair with a sleek, light-reflecting quality. It also contains rich conditioners that offer thermal protection from blow-drying and straightening.

NICKY CLARKE HAIROMATHERAPY HYDRATING SLEEK AND SHINE SERUM
Best for unruly hair
£6.49 for 75ml
The extracts of lime and orange this serum contains are there to impart dazzling shine. Here is a luxurious style finisher that gets to grips with wild hair, taming it into a sleek style; it's perfect for adding those last-minute touches that give hair that professional finish.

PAUL MITCHELL GLOSS DROPS
Best for long-lasting shine
£9.99 for 100ml

This is the product to pick if you're after shine with real staying power. It's a polishing gel that adds frizz-free definition to all hair types. Hair is left with a silky-smooth finish that lasts all day and all night.

SPACE NK HAIR GROOMING SERUM
Best for a sleek finish
£12 for 60ml

This product, suitable for all hair types, has become one of the staples in the session stylist's tool kit since it was launched two years ago. It provides a smooth, groomed finish to any look and is especially good at finishing off longer styles. Simply drop a little serum into your hand, rub your palms together and then run your hands through your hair after styling.

TERAX SHINE LOTION
Best for fine hair
£13.50 for 200ml

This lemon-infused lotion helps to restore silkiness and gloss to even the most damaged hair, leaving it soft and easy to comb through. Unlike many shine products, it doesn't weigh down your hair, but leaves it full of body.

TIGI BEDHEAD HEADRUSH SHINE ADRENALINE
Best for defining highlights
£11.50 for 100ml

A superfine, supershine mist imparting a wonderful sheen to all hair types, and particularly good for bringing out the depth and texture of highlighted hair. A few light spritzes after styling and you are ready to go.

TIGI BEDHEAD SHINE JUNKIE
Best for thick hair
£7.90 for 50ml

This is an unusual creamy polish that gives hair tremendous shine, without leaving it feeling heavy or greasy. Scoop some out with your fingers, rub it between your palms, then run through your hair to banish frizz. Its delicate fruity scent leaves hair sweet-smelling.

TONI AND GUY SHINE ZONE SPRAY
Best for long hair
£7.99 for 100ml

A little of this fine spray will add a sparkling sheen to the surface of hair, leaving it looking vibrant and healthy and smelling refreshed. It is ideal for adding shine to the drier ends of long hair, however avoid spraying it directly onto the roots as this can make long hair look lank and greasy.

TREVOR SORBIE PROFESSIONAL SERUM
Best for lifeless hair
£6.49 for 30ml
This shine serum will refresh lacklustre locks – and bring them a much-needed gloss too. You can also use it to create definition in hair that is looking a little flat. All you have to do when you apply it is to tweak individual strands to separate them from the hairstyle and add texture.

UMBERTO GIANNINI GLOSS CLOTH
Best for instant shimmer
99p for one cloth
A handbag essential that is perfect for those office-to-party nights, this buffing cloth adds immediate gloss to hair. Just smooth it all over, concentrating on dull sections, such as damaged ends or root frizz, to create dazzling shine.

UMBERTO GIANNINI MORE THAN SERUM
Best for curly hair
£6.95 for 75ml
This is the perfect product to use if you want to transform wild curls into glossy waves and ringlets. Just one pump provides enough to separate and define hair, so you're left with beautiful, frizz-free curls.

HAIRSPRAYS

AVEDA AIR-O-SOL WITCH HAZEL MEDIUM HOLD HAIR SPRAY
Best botanical hairspray
£16 for 400ml
This is the first air-powered system to disperse a fine mist of plant-based hairspray for a medium hold without stiffness or flaking. A natural UV filter and antioxidants help to prevent damage from environmental factors.

CHARLES WORTHINGTON RESULTS INVISIBLE HOLD THICKENING HAIRSPRAY
Best hairspray for fine hair
£3.99 for 200ml
This versatile spray gives subtle hold with added bounce, producing glossy styles that stay in shape for hours. Use it simply to finish a style, or, for even more volume, spray on the roots of damp hair before blow-drying.

CLINIQUE NON-AEROSOL HAIRSPRAY
Best hairspray for sensitive scalps
£10 for 237ml
Environmentally friendly and fragrance-free, this fine, clear mist gives lasting hold without making hair stiff or sticky, and it leaves very little build-up. It imparts hair

with a silky shine and brushes out easily, plus it contains conditioners to prevent hair from becoming dehydrated. Use it sparingly for a natural look.

FUDGE SKYSCRAPER MEGA HOLD HAIR LACQUER
Best hairspray for maintaining height
£6.95 for 600ml

If it's height you're after, this is the hairspray you've been looking for. It even keeps hard-to-control hair in shape and gives it lots of volume. It contains a combination of resins and conditioners which means that even styled hair stays soft to the touch, that even elaborate styles can be easily brushed out at night – and that there is no lasting brittleness.

L'OREAL ELNETT HAIRSPRAY
Best for all hair types
£3.69 for 200ml

This 40-year-old styling classic is ultra-fine, adding texture and strong, invisible hold to any style – which is why it has endured for so long and why it has endeared itself, during that time, to celebrities and hairdressers alike. Available in seven variants, it contains a satin conditioner that softens hair and improves manageability, and UV filters to protect hair from sun damage.

MICHAELJOHN VOLUME HOLD HAIRSPRAY
Best hairspray for volume
£3.99 for 250ml

As well as offering firm hold, this hairspray guarantees fuller hair with more body and swing. It contains soothing aromatherapy oils of lavender, patchouli, juniper and camomile, for fresh-smelling locks. It gives a professional 'just left the salon' finish to most hairstyles.

NEXXUS DZMAXXIMUM SUPER HOLD STYLING AND FINISHING SPRAY
Best hairspray for maximum hold
£8.90 for 400ml

The ultimate high-performance hairspray, this has incredible styling power, which makes it ideal for sculptured styles. A few spritzes of this fast-drying mist will hold most types of hair in place all day. Despite its strength it doesn't leave hair stiff or sticky and can be used daily without causing build-up.

NICKY CLARKE HAIROMATHERAPY TOTALLY TOUCHABLE HAIRSPRAY
Best hairspray for flexible hold
£4.29 for 200ml

Go for this great product if you want your hair to stay in place all day, but still feel like hair when you touch it! After a light spray, hair keeps its natural movement and bounce while aromatherapy oils protect the hair and keep it smelling fresh.

PHILOSOPHY HOLD THAT THOUGHT
Best hairspray for frizzy hair
£12.50 for 200ml
This styling spray is designed to combat frizz but is enriched with vitamins to ensure that hair is kept healthy in the process. It doesn't flake and won't dull hair with residue, instead adding shine and hold.

SPACE NK HANDBAG HAIRSPRAY
Best travel hairspray
£7.50 for 60ml
This gentle hairspray in a dinky container gives natural hold and shine to most styles – without stickiness. Suitable for all hair types, it brushes out easily, leaving hair clean and soft, with no flaky residue.

WELLA SILVIKRIN FLEXIBLE HOLD HAIRSPRAY
Best hairspray for a natural finish
£1.89 for 200ml
This light hairspray can be used to achieve a more relaxed, natural finish, leaving hair soft and supple. It also adds volume without stickiness. Ideal for fine or flyaway hair that requires gentle control.

WELLA SILVIKRIN MAXIMUM HOLD HAIRSPRAY
Best hairspray for controlled and structured styles
£1.89 for 200ml
This is a well-priced spray for strong hold without the helmet effect. It will keep a style in place for up to 24 hours and adds shine. Ideal for medium or coarse hair that demands firm control, or for short, structured styles that need added height.

HOME HAIR COLOURANTS

CHARLES WORTHINGTON DREAM COLOUR
Best colourant for glossy locks
£8.95 for one application
This product gives intense colour and exceptional shine that enhances your natural hair colour. What's more, this easy-to-use colour kit conditions your hair at the same time. There are nine shades in the range.

CLAIROL HERBAL ESSENCES HAIR COLOUR
Best ammonia-free colour
£6.95 for one application
Even though it provides intense, lasting colour, this product doesn't contain ammonia so it's gentle on your hair. And unlike most hair colourants, this one actually smells good, too, because it contains the same distinctive base fragrance as the well-known Herbal Essences shampoo range. Choose from 20 shades.

CLAIROL NICE 'N' EASY
Best treatment for long-lasting colour
£5.29 for one application
Although this permanent colour works actively with the hair's 'own tones and highlights to produce a natural look, it does cover grey completely. It contains an active conditioner for shine and creates a rich blend of colour, with plenty of depth. Choose from 32 shampoo-in shades.

CONTRASTS CHUNKY CREAM HIGHLIGHTS
Best product for a streaky effect
£6.99 for one application
Create chunky blonde streaks by simply dipping the clip-comb into the mixture and applying it to the hair you want to be blonde. It's ammonia-free and contains wheat proteins to condition the hair, plus UV filters to protect from the sun.

DANIEL GALVIN EXCLUSIVE PERMANENT COLOUR
Best colourant for natural-looking colour
£9.99 for one application
This range of colourants is designed to compliment your natural hair and eye colouring, which tends to produce a more naturalistic result. Each pack features an easy-to-use guide, so it's simple to pick the right shade. The formula contains fruit oils and jojoba, which condition the hair as it colours. Choose from 12 shades.

FUDGE PAINTBOX
Best product for funky, bright colours
£6.95 for one application
This range of semi-permanent vegetable colours caters for both the fearless and the faint-hearted. It comprises 14 bright rainbow shades from primary red to deep indigo which can be used to give a subtle tint to natural hair, or full-on vividness to pre-lightened hair. The effects last for up to ten washes.

GARNIER LUMIA BRIGHTENING COLOUR CREME
Best treatment for soft colour
£5.99 for one application
Lumia's light-reflecting technology works with the hair's natural colour to give permanent soft tones and plenty of gloss. Its cream formula contains rich natural moisturizers, such as honey and flower extracts. Choose from 20 shades.

ICE SPIKER COLORZ
Best product for metallic streaks
£7.95 for 50ml
This innovative styling glue comes in 24 sizzling shades, including some striking metallics. It's great for adding a hint of colour to spikes and layers and creating bold streaks and can be washed out the next day. It can be applied with your fingertips and is best used on dry hair.

L'OREAL EXCELLENCE CREME
Best treatment for covering grey
£7.29 for one application
The world's bestselling home hair colourant: more than 104 million packs are sold worldwide each year. The reason why it's so popular? It's fantastic for covering grey hair. What's more, it contains rich conditioners, so even fine or fragile hair can be treated without being damaged. Available in 20 colours.

L'OREAL FERIA IRIDESCENT
Best colourant for blondes
£6.99 for one application
If you want to go blonde but don't want flat, all-over colour, this is the ideal product. It gives shimmering, permanent colour, but with highlights and lowlights so that your hair has more depth and texture. The fact that the colour takes quickly is an advantage, too. Available in three light blonde shades.

L'OREAL OPEN COLOUR
Best product for disguising regrowth
£6.99 for one application
An innovative permanent colour product, this brightens your true hair colour, giving a vibrant but natural look. It enhances your natural highlights, leaving hair with a beautifully sun-kissed look. Best of all, because it's so sheer, you don't get any visible root regrowth. Choose from 20 shades.

NICKY CLARKE COLOUR
Best colourant for salon results
£7.99 for one application
The 15 semi-permanent colours in this range produce really good salon-standard results that last for 15 to 20 washes. Choose from colours such as Liquorice for dark hair and Caramel for buttery blondes. The formula contains honey and beeswax, which help infuse hair with moisture and give a glossy finish.

UMBERTO GIANNINI COLOUR LIGHTS
Best product for subtle highlights
£10.99 for one application
A genuinely easy to use, three-step highlight system that allows you to add natural-looking highlights where you choose, giving hair texture and depth, or if you just want a few strands in the front section of your hair for a sun-kissed look.

WELLA VIVA COLOUR MOUSSE
Best product for speedy results
£3.99 for one application
This mousse will add vibrant depth and shine to your colour in just 20 minutes. And because the colour lasts for only six to eight washes, it doesn't matter if you're unhappy with the result – you can soon change it. Choose from 12 shades.

HAIRBRUSHES AND COMBS

AVEDA PADDLE BRUSH
Best brush for giving volume to longer styles
£16.50
Originally created to use with scalp treatments and detangling, this professional brush features an extended-bristle design that stimulates the scalp and adds texture at the roots, for greater volume. Its gentle action reduces stress to the hair while blow-drying and styling.

CERAMIC CLAM STRAIGHTENING BRUSH
Best brush for frizz-free hair
£12.95
Set with natural bristles, this brush is brilliant for preventing frizz and static. It has ceramic-coated plates, like some top-of-the-range heated straighteners, which transfer the dryer's heat to smooth the hair cuticles and impart shine as you dry.

CHARLES WORTHINGTON IN FASHION CURLING BRUSH
Best brush for curling
£8
With a metal core, this brush heats up when you blow-dry to add body and curls to medium and long hair. The firm bristles make it perfect for turning ends either under or out and adding bounce to all hair types.

CHARLES WORTHINGTON IN FASHION ROLLERBRUSH
Best brush for versatility
£10.95
This unique brush has three detachable rollers, which can be used to set your style, add curls and waves, or give lift and volume top your roots, depending on what style or look you're after. A versatile brush that's good for all hair types.

DENMAN CLASSIC STYLER
Best brush for normal hair
£7.25
The smooth, round-ended nylon bristles of this brush are set on springy rubber cushions, making it great for shaping, smoothing and polishing all hair types. It's anti-static and is an ideal blow-drying tool.

DENMAN PADDLE BRUSH
Best brush for smooth styles
£7.95
This well-designed brush is great for serious detangling and for smoothing unruly hair. Its ball-tipped, nylon bristles prevent hair damage and help give maximum glide. Ideal for defuzzing, as it helps spread the hair's natural oils down the hair shaft, creating oodles of shine.

ERGO CONTROL BRUSH
Best brush for easy drying
£5.49

This brush makes styling surprisingly easy. The handle is designed to prevent stress on the wrist joint and can be held without awkward arm movements, so you can create the look you want with minimum effort. With anti-static bristles, it's great for faster, more accurate styling.

FREDERIC FEKKAI TECHNICIAN BRUSH
Best brush for creating waves
£30

New York-based cult hairdresser Frèdèric Fekkai designed this brush specifically to help create soft, 1940s-style, glamorous waves when blow-drying. It retains heat from the dryer, acting like a hot roller, and has nylon bristles to grip the hair well. It works especially well on fine hair.

KENT VOLUMIZING BRUSH
Best brush for creating volume
£6.95

This wide-vent brush has ball-tipped nylon bristles, which protect your hair and help decrease static. It's great for speed-drying if you're in a hurry, and adds masses of volume and body. Good for all hair types, particularly long and layered styles.

MASON PEARSON EXTRA LARGE SIZE BRISTLE BRUSH
Best brush for thick hair
£52

The crème de la crème of hair brushes. Eight oval rings of extra-stiff pure boar bristle, set in a flexible rubber cushion, provide strong but gentle brushing power. Ideal for medium-to-long, thick or wiry hair, it comes with a special cleaning attachment to help remove old hair and keep the brush in tip-top condition.

MASON PEARSON PURE BRISTLE POCKET BRISTLE BRUSH
Best handbag-size brush
£20

How often have you wanted to carry a hairbrush in your handbag, only to find that there's no room left? This handy brush by Mason Pearson – who've been making hairbrushes for 100 years – is made from pure bristle and measures just 18 cm (7 in) in length, so it will fit neatly into most bags.

MASON PEARSON TAIL COMB
Best comb for fine hair
£10

Every tooth of this great comb has been specially polished to eliminate any rough edges, which makes it excellent for styling fine, delicate hair, or teasing any hair type to new heights!

PENHALIGON'S FAUX TORTOISESHELL HAIRBRUSH
Best brush for dressing-table glamour
£125

This beautiful pure bristle brush is fabulous for thick hair, and while the handle may only be faux (fake) tortoiseshell it still oozes old-fashioned glamour and luxury. What is more, for the ultimate personal touch, Penhaligon's can arrange for your initial to be engraved on the brush. This may be a pricey purchase, but it's worth spending the money for a special gift or indulgence.

VOGUETI RAKE COMB
Best comb for wet hair
£1.99

Because wet hair is more fragile, using a brush on it can lead to breakages and split ends. This wide-toothed comb solves the problem by gently detangling and separating hair without doing any damage. It's also great for combing treatments or conditioners through hair.

HAIRDRYERS

BABYLISS DRY AND SHINE IONIC 2,000-WATT
Best hairdryer for shine
£28

This innovative, lightweight hairdryer uses 'Ion Shine' technology to generate a stream of negative ions that surround each hair, removing static electricity and smoothing the cuticles to give a shiny, conditioned finish. It has two heat settings and two speed settings, a cool-shot button and it comes with a gentle soft-finger diffuser (with soft prongs) for lift, curl and texture, a thermal straightening brush, four Velcro rollers and a pre-styling comb.

BABYLISS WHISPER JET MAX 2,400-WATT
Best hairdryer for sleek styles
£28

A megapowerful hairdryer that has three heat settings and two speed settings, as well as a concentrator nozzle for a smooth finish. Depending on what you are doing and how fast you are having to work, you can choose between two modes: Max Power, using all 2,400 watts for fast drying, or Max Quiet, which uses only 1,800 watts for quieter work.

BRAUN FUTURPRO 2,000-WATT
Best hairdryer for speed drying
£22.99

If it's an extra ten minutes in bed each morning you're after, this is the dryer for you – hair dries in around half the usual time. There are three heat and two speed settings, making it easy to adjust to meet your styling needs.

CHARLES WORTHINGTON PERFORMANCE TI TURBO 2,000-WATT
Best budget-buy hairdryer
Around £19.99

This lightweight but powerful design offers 2,000-watt drying performance for speedy styling. It's hard-wearing, scratch-resistant metallic finish helps to protect it from wear and tear and makes it a stylish addition to any dressing table.

MORPHY RICHARDS MARK HILL POWER DRY 2,400-WATT
Best hairdryer for ultimate power
£24.99

One of the most powerful hairdryers on the market, this gives extremely professional results. It has an adjustable nozzle that enables you to control the airflow. Setting the nozzle to the narrow positions allows you to get hair dead straight, while opening it wider increases the airflow for a more tousled look.

MORPHY RICHARDS VOYAGER TRAVEL 800-WATT
Best hairdryer for weekends away
£7.99

Small, and yet with plenty of power, this is perfect for when you're away from home for a few days. It folds easily in half for compact storage, and, despite its size, manages to provide two heat and two speed settings.

OPAL MARVELLOUS MINI
Best hairdryer for international travel
£9.99

At a mere 11cm x 5.5cm (4 $\frac{1}{2}$ x 2in) when folded, this is possibly the smallest hairdryer available. It has two speed settings and a dual-voltage switch to ensure that it can be used safely in any country. You can choose from four pastel colours – sea green, baby blue, peach and white – and it comes with a carrying pouch.

PHILIPS OPTIVOLUME SUPER SILENCE 1,800-WATT
Best hairdryer for quiet drying
£20

This light, compact hairdryer comes with both a diffuser for curly styles and a concentrator nozzle for sleeker looks. Best of all, it's very quiet compared to the average hairdryer, so you'll still be able to listen to the radio as you dry your hair!

TIPS

- Don't rub your hair when you are towel-drying – blot it dry gently or else you may risk damaging it.
- Never brush wet hair; instead, comb it through with a wide-tooth comb.
- Always allow your hair to dry a little before blow-drying it and make sure that the dryer is not too hot.

REMINGTON TOTAL PERFORMANCE RETRO 2,000-WATT
Best durable hairdryer
£22.99
Boasting four heat settings, two speed settings and a cool-shot button, this powerful hairdryer will leave you with hair that looks as though you've just walked out of the salon. It also features a dust-guard filter system that keeps out fluff.

VIDAL SASSOON HAIR HYDRATION 1,800-WATT
Best hairdryer for damaged hair
£29.99
This hairdryer is good for preventing the heat damage that can occur when you use a hairdryer every day, and produces salon-smooth results. It releases negative ions, which help to moisturize and reduce frizziness, leaving hair glossy and static-free.

VIDAL SASSOON MAXIMUM FUNK IT UP 2,000-WATT
Best hairdryer for funky styles
£19.99
This low-noise hairdryer has a multifunction nozzle for either a choppy style or smooth-looking hair. The twisting handle has three different holding positions and Vidal Sassoon Defining Wax is supplied to help you to create the look you want.

WIGO TAIFUN PROFESSIONAL ORIGINAL CHROME 1,000-WATT
Best-looking hairdryer
£45
This is a truly chic-looking dryer, which has made it the all-time favourite of many session stylists. Its classic chrome design is matched by its power, two heat and two speed combinations, and a cold shot to set hair.

HAIR STRAIGHTENERS

BABYLISS PRO CERAMIC STRAIGHTENERS
Best for thick hair
£48.50
A high-quality tool, this is specially designed for the demands of professional salon use. The slimline, ceramic-coated plates are cleverly sprung to self-adjust to the thickness of your hair, ensuring you never get gaps between the plates. It produces amazing results and is incredibly easy to use.

BABYLISS STRAIGHT 'N' SHINE PLUS
Best for shine
£20
This straightener uses a gentle steam mist to protect hair and add shine while it straightens, for glossy locks. It also has a removable detangling comb for pre-styling, and is multivoltage for worldwide use.

BRAUN STEAM AND STRAIGHT BSS
Best for holidays
£23.99

This cordless styler is ideal for getting long hair dead straight. It heats up quickly but the procedure is gentle, because it emits a shot of steam to put moisture back into hair, as it sets it for a long-lasting look. It is compact enough to take anywhere.

CARMEN REAL SMOOTHIE STRAIGHTENER
Best easy-to-use straightener
£19.99

This dinky, disc-shaped gadget fits snugly into the palm of your hand, so that you can run it easily through your hair. A steam facility means that it protects your hair from heat damage; it adds moisture and shine as it smoothes.

DANAMATIC IRON
Best for Afro hair
£48

These professional straightening irons are heavy duty enough to cope with any hair texture, making them ideal to use on Afro hair. Remarkably, they leave the hair shiny and frizz-free.

DANIEL HERSHESON STRAIGHTENING IRONS
Best for a professional finish
£80

These irons have become a beauty icon – Jennifer Aniston and Elle Macpherson (regulars at the celebrity salon) are both said to be big fans. The jumbo-size plates mean there's no easier, quicker method of straightening hair at home, leaving it with incredible shine.

GHD HAIR STYLING IRON
Best for damaged hair
£87.50

The ultimate in hair straightening, these irons heat up in six seconds! They're computer-chip powered for constant, even heat monitoring, giving you full control as you style. As well as ceramic plates, they have a ceramic heating element to produce a negative ion charge that seals in moisture, natural oils and hair colour, creating fantastic shine with minimum damage.

HAIR ART INTERNATIONAL HAIR STIK
Best for colour-treated hair
£79.50

These straigheners are America's bestselling ceramic irons. They incorporate ultra-fast heating, adjustable heat control and supersmooth plates – to suit all hair types. The 2.5 cm (1 in) plates are specially coated to protect hair and lock in moisture, thereby helping to prevent damage to colour-treated hair.

MORPHY RICHARDS MARK HILL MOBILE STRAIGHTENER
Best multipurpose travel straightener
£29.99

For great hair on the go, this tube-shaped, chrome-finished straightener is perfect. It's designed to be rechargeable from either the mains or a car cigarette lighter and to provide 30 minutes of continued use. A handbag essential for nights out after work and ideal, too, for slipping into a suitcase.

NICKY CLARKE PROFESSIONAL SLIM STRAIGHTENER NCS6
Best for fringes
£19.99

These 12 mm ($1/2$ in) scissor-action straighteners are ideal for shorter hair and great if you want to smooth fringes and individual sections. The matt black, ultra-glide coated plates leave short hair shiny and sleek.

REMINGTON SUPER SMOOTH PROFESSIONAL STRAIGHTENER
Best for very curly hair
£29.99

This professional straightener works wonders on wayward hair; its high temperatures necessary for getting hair perfectly straight – fast! It has large, Teflon-coated plates that not only prevent static but also help your hair to glide smoothly through. This implement has a lightweight handle, which makes it easy to hold and not too tiring to use.

REMINGTON SUPER STEAM STRAIGHTENER C1100
Best for versatility
£24.99

For the Nicole Kidmans among us, who sometimes go straight but sometimes want curls, this tool uses steam to smooth out waves and create glossiness, while Teflon-coated plates glide easily through all hair types, preventing static, stickiness and hairspray build-up. Waving and crimping plates increase your options.

SLEEKER CONVEX CERAMIC STYLER
Best for fine hair
£69.95

The tiny plates clamp together tightly to hold and straighten even the finest hair, and they are really good for flicking up the ends. By creating negative ions, they also seal in the moisture, thereby protecting delicate hair.

VIDAL SASSOON MINI STRAIGHTEN IT OUT
Best handbag straightener
£21.99

This handy gadget is small enough to take on holiday, or for a weekend away. And it has a variable temperature gauge, so you can minimize heat damage and won't need to worry about frying your locks. Available in chrome and black.

CURLING APPLIANCES

BABYLISS TREVOR SORBIE PROFESSIONAL SESSION CURLING IRONS
Best for dry hair
£17

These mid-size steam tongs give long-lasting curls and waves. The gentle steam mist can be used at the press of a button and helps add shine to damaged or delicate hair. They come with a brush attachment and four metal sectioning clips for more precise styling.

BRAUN INDEPENDENT STEAM C80S
Best cordless curler
£24.99

Recently made available in lilac, this handy tool works on a 14g gas cartridge, which makes it the perfect choice for when you're on the move. The curling tong is ideal for spiral curls, while the styling brush is like a giant roller, creating soft waves. It also features a shot of steam, a shaping brush for extra body and two sectioning clips to help you style more easily.

CARMEN 4U CURL UP STEAM ROLLERS
Best for soft curls
£29.99

A classic in hair styling, these rollers were created in 1966 by an entrepreneur who wanted to make something to help curl his wife's stubbornly straight hair. The steam facility helps to set the style, while maintaining the hair's natural shine. The set comes with 12 large rollers, eight smaller ones and 20 butterfly clips. Lasting volume, lift or curl is the result.

DANIEL HERSHESON WAVING TONGS
Best for professional waves
£70

For natural-looking waves, simply wrap hair section by section around the curved part of these tongs, clinch together and release. Daniel himself recommends making your own setting lotion by dissolving 2 tbsp salt and 1 tsp sugar in half a pint of water – he swears it works better than shop-bought products.

MORPHY RICHARDS MARK HILL CRIMP MATES
Best crimper
£27.99

If you're crazy for crimped hair, look no further than this gadget. It has three interchangeable plates to create different looks, whatever your mood. There's a crimping plate, a straightening plate and a box-crimping plate, which makes big, funky waves. It also has rubberized finger-grips at the end of each plate so you won't burn your fingers.

MORPHY RICHARDS MARK HILL STYLE IT HOT AIR STYLER
Best for curling as you dry
£24.99

This 800-watt appliance enables you to dry and curl hair at the same time. It comprises two Velcro brushes for curl and a brush designed to counteract static, and even a diffuser for achieving volume. There are three heat settings and a cool-shot button to help set your impressive results.

NICKY CLARKE TWIST AND SHAPE SLIM SALON TONG
Best for spiral curls
£13.99

An ultra-slim tong that creates beautiful spiral-shape curls, this has two settings: high for thick hair and low for fine or short hair. Simply wind your hair around it, then hold in place for five to 15 seconds. Although it's a bit fiddly to use at first, the spectacular results make persevering until you get the hang of it worthwhile. It's also ideal for curling any dangling tendrils when hair is put up.

PHILIPS GEOMETRICS STYLER
Best for versatility
£23

The ultimate gadget for women who like to change their minds, it has six attachments to give you every style you could possibly desire. Flirt with two different-width curling tongs, a spiral tong, a brush, a straightener and a crimper.

REMINGTON BIG SHOT POWER STYLER
Best for quick curls
£26.99

This 1000-watt airstyler has the power to persuade poker-straight locks into curls in double-quick time. Use the large, round brush to add volume, the slimmer round brush to create curls and the straightening head for flicking out ends. The hot-air function means that it can double as a hairdryer.

REMINGTON FLEXI CURLS
Best for cascading curls
£29.99

These flexible heated curlers are ideal for creating corkscrew curls in long hair. The 20 twisting rollers have a self-locking mechanism and change colour when it's time to take them out. Perfect if you're looking to create the Pre-Raphaelite look.

TIGI HARDCORE WAVE RUNNER
Best for sculpted waves
£45

Easy to use and incorporating a temperature control so that you don't fry your hair for too long, this innovative triple-barrelled curling iron is perfect for creating soft 'gypsy' waves in medium to long hair.

Fragrance is the ultimate sensory experience. It can make you feel happy, nostalgic, refreshed or sensual. The scent you choose to wear is very personal, not least because skin reacts in a unique way to each scent. What smells great on your best friend may not suit you.

Today there are over 1,100 different fragrances available, which makes choosing the right one for you somewhat perplexing! And despite being one of the most expensive beauty purchases you'll make, two-thirds of the fragrances we buy remain in the box, untouched. Therefore, its important to understand a few basic rules.

The difference between perfume, eau de parfum, eau de toilette and eau de cologne depends on the amount of oils present in the fragrance: the higher the concentration of oils, the longer the fragrance will last. Perfume contains the highest, next comes eau de parfum, then eau de toilette and finally eau de cologne. A fragrance is comprised of different scents, which are referred to as 'notes'. Top notes are extremely light and are what you smell when you first apply the scent. They usually last for only a few minutes. Middle notes take longer to develop and are noticeable after about 15 minutes. These notes tend to last for about an hour. Base notes are the stronger ingredients and last the longest, usually several hours.

Fragrances belong to one of six main fragrance families: floral, chypre/woody, fougère, oriental, citrus or ozonic, or combinations of these. Traditionally, floral and citrus fragrances are recommended for daytime or casual wear, while spicy, woody or warmer-based scents are thought more suitable for the evening. These days, however, people tend to be more daring with scent and wear what they like, when they like. And while in the past women often had a 'signature scent' – one fragrance they always wore – most women today own several fragrances and alternate between them. It would be impossible to list all the fragrances that are available today but this chapter has tried to include some of the most popular ones.

FRAGRANCE FAMILIES

Floral: Soft, feminine and easy to wear, floral is the most popular family. Ranging from single notes to heady bouquets, they include rose, lily of the valley, freesia and violet.

Chypre/Woody: The term 'chypre' comes from the first significant mossy-wood fragrance, Chypre de Coty, created by François Coty in 1917. Redolent of oakmoss, sandalwood and musk, these notes are often combined with jasmine, rose or citrus.

Fougère: This family originated from the release of Houbigant's aromatic Fougère Royale in 1882, and has come to have universal appeal. Often unisex, these are an eclectic mix of citrus, lavender and oriental notes with sweet spices.

Oriental: Full of warmth, these combine woods, spices, musk and amber with citrus, green or fruity top notes to create sultry and seductive scents. Orientals can be heavy, but they are also long-lasting.

Citrus: Crisp and refreshing, the zest of lemons, oranges, grapefruit and bergamot oils gives these scents their unique tangy aroma.

Ozonic: The latest addition, ozonics emerged in the 1990s with the discovery of aroma chemicals that could impart the scent of wet air and the seaside. These water notes are often used to enhance floral, oriental and woody fragrances.

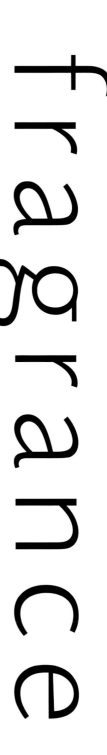

fragrance

CHANEL – CHANCE
Variable floral
Eau de parfum, £35 for 50ml

The revolutionary spherical construction of Chanel's new fragrance means that whereas, traditionally, a perfume is characterized by a succession of notes, in this case the dominant scent of the fragrance is perpetually changing. Because Chance not only contains hyacinth, jasmine, fresh vetiver, absolute of iris, pink pepper, white musk, citrus and amber of patchouli and also contains a secret element that Chanel describes as 'the unexpected accord which gives it its life and vitality', this fragrance cannot really be labelled as belonging to any particular fragrance group.

FLORAL

ALESSANDRO DELL'ACQUA – ALESSANDRO DELL'ACQUA
Spicy floral
Eau de toilette, £30 for 50ml; £45 for 100ml

A unique and deeply sensual floral-musk fragrance, which is powerful and yet, at the same time, subtle. Distinctive top notes of pelargonium, lathyrus and coriander open the scent, warming to a delicate heart of rose, peony and hibiscus. Soft base notes of sandalwood, musk and incense then blend to create a rich, enveloping finish.

ANNICK GOUTAL – GRAND AMOUR
Rich floral
Eau de toilette, £39 for 50ml

A sexy, floral to wear every day. Gentle top notes of peony, rose and geranium are released first, enhanced by a fruity middle of redcurrants, pomegranates, cherries and peaches. A base of musk and cedarwood adds warmth and richness.

ANTONIA'S FLOWERS – ANTONIA'S FLOWERS
Crisp floral
Eau de toilette, £38 for 50ml

One of New York's favourite fragrances, this is a light, fresh and subtle scent based on the creator's favourite flowers, freesias, which she blends with notes of lily, magnolia, jasmine and sandalwood. The result smells just like fresh-cut flowers.

CACHAREL – ANAIS ANAIS
Fresh floral
Eau de toilette, £28 for 50ml; £44 for 100ml

This sweet floral classic is ideal for daytime. A fresh burst of hyacinth in this fragrance melts into soft orange blossom and then mingles with a heady heart of jasmine, iris and rose absolute. The muskiness of cedar, sandalwood and vetiver adds lasting depth.

CALVIN KLEIN – ETERNITY
Fresh floral

Eau de toilette, £35 for 50ml; £52 for 100ml

Launching this fragrance in 1988, Calvin Klein described it as the embodiment of 'romance with commitment'. Freesia, lily, lily of the valley and narcissus fuse with mandarin, sandalwood and wild flowers in a clean, soft, enduringly romantic scent.

CARON – BLACK NARCISSUS
Rich floral

Eau de parfum, £44 for 50ml

Silent-screen legend Gloria Swanson was quick to make this perfume, created in 1911, her signature scent. It has a sumptuous top note of orange blossom and daffodil that moves into a heady heart of rose, jasmine and orange. The lingering base is comprised of sandalwood, musk and vetiver.

CARON – FLEURS DE ROCAILLE
Crisp floral

Eau de parfum, £45 for 50ml

A simple yet captivating perfume that opens with fragrant gardenia and violet top notes. Next comes the heart of rich florals including lily of the valley, jasmine, lilac and mimosa, culminating in a vibrant base of cedar, sandalwood and amber.

CAUDALIE – FLEUR DE VIGNE
Fruity floral

Eau fraiche energisante, £31 for 100ml

From the French Vinothérapie company, Caudalie, this unique fragrance is based on the vine flower – a small white bloom that signals the start of the grape harvest. The top note is green and floral with hints of freesia and lily of the valley; the heart is light but satisfying. Dry cedar and a drop of sandalwood are at the base.

CHANEL – CHANEL NO.5
Classic soft floral

Eau de parfum, £48 for 50ml

This iconic classic was the first perfume created by Coco Chanel and the first to bear a designer's name. Marilyn Monroe famously claimed that it was all that she wore in bed. Its first notes are mixed, light florals, including ylang ylang and neroli, although these are quickly followed by a heady centre of rose and jasmine. There is a lingering base of sandalwood and vetiver which gives a vibrant, woody finish.

CHANEL – CHANEL NO.19
Woody floral

Eau de parfum, £48 for 50ml

Created in 1970, this daring but delicate perfume has become a favourite. It opens with neroli and galbanum, perfectly complemented by the powerful floral heart of iris, narcissus and rose. The base of rich cedar and moss emphasizes its strength.

CHANTECAILLE – LE JASMINE DE CHANTECAILLE
Rich floral

Eau de parfum, £69 for 50ml; £110 for 100ml

This delightful concoction captures the intense and intoxicating scent of jasmine flowers. It really is a true indulgence because, for every ounce of fragrance created, 36,000 flowers are needed, making it the most expensive flower perfume in existence. Beginning with fresh notes of mimosa and magnolia, the middle is composed of a pure jasmine, strengthened by tuberose. A touch of oak moss and amber provide depth at the base.

CHLOE – NARCISSE
Oriental floral

Eau de toilette, £31 for 50ml; £42.50 for 75ml

An intense floral that is suitable for day or evening wear. The top notes include delicate frangipani, apricot, marigold and orange blossom, warming to a rich heart of jasmine, rose and Eastern spices. Further depth is introduced with a sensual mix of sandalwood, vanilla and musk.

CHRISTIAN DIOR – ADDICT
Fresh oriental floral

Eau de parfum, £39 for 50ml; £55 for 100ml

Sexy, strong and edgier than any of its Dior predecessors, Addict is ideal for evenings out. Top notes of mandarin leaf and silk-tree flower introduce the fragrance with freshness, before the strong impact of queen of the night – a rare, vanilla-scented flower that grows in Jamaica. Rose and jasmine then fill and round out the floral heart, the base notes of Bourbon vanilla, sandalwood and tonka bean adding further intensity at the finish.

CHRISTIAN DIOR – DIORISSIMO
Fresh floral

Eau de toilette, £36.50 for 50ml

A distinctively feminine blend with its foundations in the delicate scent of lily of the valley, this fragrance is perfect for daytime wear. After the first notes – a mixture of freshly crushed lily leaves and ylang ylang – the fragrance unfolds into the full scent of the little lily, before its rounded conclusion, a warm and rich sensuous note of jasmine.

CHRISTIAN DIOR – J'ADORE
Fresh floral

Eau de toilette, £37 for 50ml; £52 for 100ml

A sparkling, fresh floral, J'Adore is sensuous, contemporary and feminine. Among the top notes are champaca flower, mandarin and ivy leaves, for a bracing first impression, but a heart of orchids, violet and rose emerges to soften the scent. That is in turn succeeded by a base comprising rich Damascus plum, amaranth wood and blackberry musk.

CLINIQUE – HAPPY
Fresh floral
Eau de toilette, £29.50 for 50ml; £42.50 for 100ml

A chic, modern fragrance that mingles vibrant citrus with floral softness. Exotically fruity top notes contain grapefruit and boysenberry that blend with the middle note of Hawaiian wedding flower. A soft cedarwood base completes the bouquet.

CREED – SPRING FLOWER
Rich floral
Eau de parfum, £39.50 for 30ml

Ideal for a summer's day, this perfume combines vibrant fresh green notes with sweet tones of melon, peach, apricot and apples intermingled with exquisite jasmine and rose. The base is of subtle, sensual musk. It's Julia Roberts's favourite.

CREED – FLEURISSIMO
Fresh floral
Eau de parfum, £39.50 for 30ml

Prince Rainier of Monaco commissioned this scent so that Grace Kelly could wear it on their wedding day and its sophisticated fragrance has secured its status as a classic ever since. Delicate rose and tuberose make up the top notes, while a delightful mixture of violet leaves and Florentine iris comprise both heart and base.

DONNA KARAN – CASHMERE MIST
Sheer floral
Eau de toilette, £37 for 50ml; £54 for 100ml

'Cashmere', insists designer Donna Karan, 'is my favourite thing to have next to my skin.' This fragrance was her way of capturing the sensual caress of this luxurious fabric. Its top notes bring together Moroccan jasmine with lily of the valley, followed by a heart of bracing bergamot. This is then enveloped in a base of warm, sultry sandalwood, amber and musk.

ESTEE LAUDER – BEAUTIFUL
Crisp floral
Eau de parfum, £30 for 30ml; £50 for 75ml

Many flowers combine to make this one of Lauder's most romantic, feminine perfumes. Vibrant rose, lily, marigold and carnation are among the complex top and middle notes, while sandalwood, vetiver and moss furnish a sensual base.

ESTEE LAUDER – PLEASURES INTENSE
Sheer floral
Eau de parfum, £34 for 50ml; £50 for 100ml

A fresh summer essential, this light floral opens with a clear, dewy top note of white lilies and violet leaves, lifted by watery accents. A deep centre follows, of black lilacs, peonies, roses and exotic karo karounde blossom, plus a tingle of peppery old French rose and then rich Indian sandalwood and patchouli linger.

ETRO – RESORT
Fruity floral
Eau de toilette, £38 for 150ml

This energizing and exotic blend of sharp citrus and summer florals is one to splash on. Top notes include lemon, lime, mandarin and grapefruit, which lead into a middle of lily, jasmine and magnolia. A subtle sandalwood and patchouli base completes the identity of this classic scent.

FRESH – PATCHOULI PURE
Rich floral
Eau de parfum, £60 for 100ml

Forget patchouli's 1960s hippy associations, this perfume is distinctly modern and sophisticated. With patchouli at its centre, each of the surrounding notes helps to bring out its unique richness: the top is characterized by invigorating ginger, orange and cinnamon while the base is a mellow vanilla, amber and musk.

GHOST – GHOST
Deep floral
Eau de toilette, £41 for 100ml

Chic and sophisticated, the top notes of rose petal and ambrette seed open and warm to a rich floral heart of pure white flowers and jasmine with incense. A fruity, sensual base of vanilla, musk, amber and apricot completes this delicate blend.

GIORGIO ARMANI – ACQUA DI GIO
Aquatic floral
Eau de toilette, £25 for 35ml

A refreshing flowery scent that blends fresh-cut flowers with cool water. Opening notes of sweet pea and the aroma of sea spray are fused with a heart of jasmine, freesia, hyacinth and muscat grape, and rounded off with a light musky base.

GIVENCHY – AMARIGE
Spicy floral
Eau de toilette, £38 for 50ml; £56 for 100ml

An intense fragrance based on a bouquet of white flowers. Crisp top notes of tangerine, violet and rosewood hit you first, followed by heady heart gardenia, mimosa and ylang ylang. Amber, musk and vanilla create a muted, yet warm, base.

TIPS

- Florals are great for spring, and citruses and ozonics are good daytime options.
- For a long-lasting effect, build up your fragrance in layers: start with the shower or bath gel and body lotion, and only then add the perfume.
- To leave your hair alluringly scented, try the hair fragrances now offered by some perfumiers.

▓ GRES – CABOTINE
Fresh floral
Eau de toilette, £25 for 50ml
Every note of this romantic scent revolves around the ginger lily. Blended with
this are the fruity notes of blackcurrant buds and mandarin, the sweet, spicy notes
of orange blossom and tuberose, and the warmth of sandalwood. It is pretty,
young and vibrant.

▓ GUERLAIN – CHAMPS ELYSEES
Fresh floral
Eau de toilette, £26 for 50ml
A fresh, radiant scent – delicate but sophisticated. Mimosa leaves and rose petals
offer gentle opening notes and blend with warmer buddleia, mimosa blossom and
blackcurrant at the heart. A base of almond wood adds a unique, lingering finish.

▓ GUY LA ROCHE – FIDJI
Fresh floral
Eau de parfum, £29.99 for 100ml
Developed in the 1960s, inspired by the imagery of a South Sea island, fresh
breezes and flowers, this perfume includes the slightly green tones of galbanum
and iris with the spicy floral tones of jasmine and rose based on musk, patchouli
and sandalwood. It is soft, fresh and flowery, and yet spicy and strong.

▓ HELMUT LANG – FOR HER
Spicy floral
Eau de parfum, £32 for 50ml
A distinctly modern, woody perfume for everyday wear. Top notes of rose,
orange tree and jasmine open, followed by a rich middle of rose and lily of the
valley. Indian sandalwood, vanilla and patchouli form the warm base.

▓ JEAN PATOU – JOY
Classic floral
Eau de toilette, £60 for 75ml
A luxurious and sophisticated scent, created in 1930 to be the 'costliest perfume
in the world'. One single ounce of Joy contains 10,600 jasmine flowers and 28
dozen roses! Top notes of rose, ylang ylang and tuberose blend with a heart of
jasmine and May rose, rounded off with warm musk at the base.

▓ JEAN-PAUL GAULTIER – FRAGILE
Spicy floral
Eau de parfum, £47 for 50ml
The rare and richly scented tuberose flower is the main constituent of this new
perfume. First impressions are of stimulating raspberry leaves and sweet orange,
then the middle is floral, emboldened by spicy capsicum and pink pepper. Base
notes enriched with cedar, musk and violet wood offer an unforgettable finale.

▇ JEAN-PAUL GAULTIER – JEAN-PAUL GAULTIER
Crisp oriental floral

Eau de parfum, £35.50 for 30ml

A fruity, sophisticated yet provocative perfume. Aromatic rum and rose enrich the top, while the middle unfolds with jonquil and rich vanilla orchid, before a sensual signature, a flourish of Bourbon vanilla, sandalwood and sweet amber.

▇ JIL SANDER – SUN FRAGRANCE
Soft floral

Eau de toilette, £15 for 30ml; £23.50 for 75ml

Created in 1989 to mimic a warm evening breeze, this refreshing, summery fragrance delicately combines top notes of bergamot and rosewood with hints of jasmine and vanilla, awakening the senses and leaving the skin beautifully scented. Unusually, it can be worn in the sun without risk of sunburn or pigmentation.

▇ KENZO – FLOWER
Soft floral

Eau de parfum, £35 for 50ml; £45 for 100ml

A powdery-floral perfume with a modern feel. The first notes unfold with Parma violet, wild hawthorn, cassia and Bulgarian rose, mingling with the warm, rich heart of vanilla and white musk. A final discreet base of hedione adds lasting freshness.

▇ LACOSTE – LACOSTE POUR FEMME
Warm floral

Eau de toilette, £29 for 50ml; £36 for 90ml

A sophisticated new fragrance from a company traditionally associated with men's aftershave. Bergamot and pepper make for a vibrant top note that builds around a heart that mixes the rare white heliotrope flower with hibiscus. The floral tones are then balanced with the muskiness of an ambrette seed base.

▇ LANVIN – ARPEGE
Rich floral

Eau de parfum, £35 for 50ml

Originally launched in 1927, then relaunched under the new ownership of the L'Oréal company in 1993, this classic perfume continues to retain the richness of its famous floral bouquet. Notes include patchouli, sandalwood, ylang ylang, rose, jasmine, lily of the valley, bergamot and aldehydes. A rich and intriguing scent.

▇ LANVIN – OXYGENE
Light floral

Eau de parfum, £36.50 for 50ml; £47 for 75ml

This radiant perfume is composed of a captivating blend of flowers and woody scents. Hyssop, a plant known for its stimulating properties, hits first, followed by a rich mix of gardenia, blue iris and sandalwood at the heart. Spicy bottom notes of white musk and white pepper then add depth.

■ MARC JACOBS – GARDENIA
Aquatic floral
Eau de parfum, £49 for 50ml; £69 for 100ml
An aquatic note with a hint of fruity bergamot opens this subtle but intoxicating perfume, before a middle of pure gardenia, accented by honeysuckle, white pepper and Egyptian jasmine, and a perfect finish of subtly blended creamy musks.

■ MILLER HARRIS – FLEUR DU MATIN
Soft floral
Eau de parfum, £48 for 100ml
This is a subtle yet enticing fragrance, classically feminine but modern, and incorporating among its ingredients lemon leaves, neroli, honeysuckle, jasmine, basil and grapefruit, evidence that its creation was inspired by perfumier Lyn Harris's trip to an island off the south of France.

■ NAJ OLEARI – NAJ OLEARI PARFUM
Spicy floral
Eau de toilette, £20 for 50ml
An extremely feminine fragrance with both floral and musk notes making it a sensual and romantic scent. Included are lily of the valley and coriander, blended with freesia and jasmine in a base of white musks, sandalwood and vanilla.

■ NINA RICCI – L'AIR DU TEMPS
Fresh floral
Eau de toilette, £24 for 30ml
Ideal for everyday wear, here is a soft, timeless classic, fondly remembered for its frosted glass bottle by Lalique. Top notes of jasmine melt into heady gardenia and carnation at the heart, enriched by a warm and sensual sandalwood base note.

■ OSCAR DE LA RENTA – INTRUSION
Warm floral
Eau de parfum, £40 for 50ml
Tangy Sicilian bergamot tangoes with the delicacy of neroli and soft star anise in the top notes of this charming perfume. The middle comprises a white bouquet – of peony, jasmine, gardenia and lily – with a touch of coriander for a subtle, spicy note. Base notes of patchouli, amber and musk give fullness and warmth.

■ PAUL SMITH – EXTREME
Light floral
Eau de toilette, £27 for 50ml; £37 for 100ml
The latest fragrant offering from designer Paul Smith is a sensuous, lively scent, with a touch of old-fashioned elegance. Fruity top notes of mandarin, blackcurrant and freesia open the scent and move into a core comprising whole blackcurrant branches, softened by violet petals. The final notes come from amber and musk with a resonance of sandalwood and cedar.

fragrances

▦ PENHALIGON'S – LOVE POTION NO.9 FOR LADIES
Rich floral
Eau de toilette, £30 for 50ml; £47 for 100ml
Soft, spicy and rich, this magical potion is designed to impart in its wearers an air of irresistibility. Top notes of cypress, neroli, lemon and mandarin awaken the senses while the middle is heady – jasmine and rose, mixed with spicy coriander and clove. Base notes of sandalwood, vanilla and tonka leave a lingering richness.

▦ RALPH LAUREN – GLAMOROUS
Spicy floral
Eau de parfum, £41 for 50ml
A sensuous and elegant new perfume with unusual notes that make it perfect for evenings. First you get clementine, pearl flower and lily, followed by a heart of ginger flower and wild tuberose. Ultimately, an exotic mixture of Siam wood, cashmere and vetiver complete the experience.

▦ RALPH LAUREN – ROMANCE
Fresh floral
Eau de toilette, £37.50 for 50ml
The top notes of this romantic scent highlight *Rosa* 'Sun Goddess' with its fresh, citrus aroma. It was this bright yellow flower – a favourite of Lauren and grown in his garden – that inspired the fragrance. The middle notes boast the warmth of lotus petals, a flower that represents the essence of love, while the bottom notes combine sensual musk, exotic woods and oak moss, creating depth and richness.

▦ REVLON – CHARLIE SILVER
Fruity floral
Eau de toilette, £8.95 for 30ml; £11.95 for 50ml
A gorgeous combination of crisp green notes with a clean, woody base. One quick spritz and you'll smell a burst of pear and green vine flower, followed by the sweet middle notes of heather, magnolia and linden tree sap. Finally, base notes of golden wood, musk and amber are unleashed and linger all day.

▦ ROCHAS – MADAME ROCHAS
Rich floral
Eau de toilette, £32 for 50ml; £51 for 100ml
A soft, feminine and refined fragrance, created in Paris in 1960. Top notes of neroli and genista open the scent, before it warms to a heart of lilac, jasmine, tuberose and orange blossom, and warm base notes of amber and sandalwood add depth.

▦ STILA – BOUQUET DU JOUR
Light floral
Eau de parfum, £36 each for 200ml
This bespoke fragrance concept enables you to customize your scent to fit your mood. It consists of two eaux de parfum: Jade Blossom, a fresh, crisp blend of

green tea, cucumber and lemon verbena, and Crème Blossom, a sweet, delicate blend of vanilla, pink lilac and lily of the valley. Both have three coordinating body lotions that each pick out a single note of the perfumes and which can be mixed in any combination for truly individual fragrance layering.

▨ SYLVIE CHANTECAILLE – DARBY ROSE
Classic floral

Eau de parfum, £59 for 50ml

English rose 'Abraham Darby' is the key ingredient of this pretty perfume, which includes base notes of vetiver, sandalwood and musk with bursts of magnolia, mandarin and lemon – lovely, charismatic blend of the old-fashioned and modern.

▨ TOMMY HILFIGER – TOMMY GIRL
Fresh floral

Eau de toilette, £26 for 50ml; £36 for 100ml

Inspired by wild flowers gathered from the American landscape, this effervescent scent is spirited and sexy. Top notes include bergamot and mandarin, while the middle combines the phlox flower with wild daffodil. Finally, a sensuous but light base of vetiver rounds off the fragrance.

▨ TRUSSARDI – SKIN
Oriental floral

Eau de parfum, £35 for 50ml
Eau de toilette, £44 for 75ml

This is a truly sensuous fragrance. Initially the fragrance seems strongly fruity but prolonged contact seems to allow it to blend with the skin so that it becomes enduringly delicate. The top notes, comprising violet leaves, bergamot and mandarin orange, seem to shimmer over a heart of rose, jasmine and lily of the valley, which then, in turn, blends with a base of patchouli, moss and chypre.

▨ VALENTINO – VALENTINO GOLD
Modern floral

Eau de parfum, £41 for 50ml; £57.50 for 100 ml

The classic designer has created a modern but distinctly feminine perfume in Gold. Fresh top notes of mandarin, key lime and cardamom soften to mellow middle notes of cranberry and ginger water lily. A vibrant bottom note of blue iris is then blended with the seductive warmth of sandalwood, cinnamon and musk, to create a long-lasting scent.

▨ VAN CLEEF & ARPELS – BIRMANE
Light floral

Eau de parfum, £45 for 50ml

A casual, girlish perfume with top notes of freesia and fruits heralding a heart of jasmine and white rose. A rich base of musk, tonka bean, cedar and red lily completes this unusual fragrance.

■ VAN CLEEF & ARPELS – FIRST
Rich soft floral
Eau de toilette, £41.50 for 60ml

Using jasmine from Grasse, Turkish rose and ylang ylang among its ingredients, as well as blackcurrant buds, mandarin and bergamot, this is the first fragrance to be created by the grand French jewellery house. Base notes of sandalwood, amber and musk ensure that it is a powerful, sophisticated and mature scent.

■ VAN CLEEF & ARPELS – MURMURE
Spicy floral
Eau de toilette, £36 for 50ml

This is a sophisticated, traditional scent with top notes of mandarin and a delicious floral blend of freesia, white rose and jasmine. Next to resonate are the warm middle notes of orange blossom and cassis flower. Then finally comes a harmony of woody scents, such as vanilla, Brazilian rosewood and cedar.

■ VERA WANG – VERA WANG
Modern floral
Eau de parfum, £68 for 100ml

A decidedly feminine perfume from the iconic queen of the bridal gown. Top notes of Bulgarian rose, mandarin flower and a floral heart of lotus and gardenia make this one of the most desirable fragrances of 2003.

■ VIVIENNE WESTWOOD – BOUDOIR
Rich floral
Eau de toilette, £30 for 30ml; £45 for 50ml

Sensual and sophisticated, top notes of white viburnum, mandarin and bergamot weave around middle notes of coriander and red roses in this louche fragrance. Base notes of vanilla, sandalwood and amber seal the affair.

■ YVES SAINT LAURENT – BABY DOLL
Fresh floral
Eau de parfum, £20 for 30ml; £30 for 50ml

A flirty, young perfume that blends spice, flowers and citrus. Top notes include fruity grapefruit, redcurrant and rhubarb, before a floral heart unfolds, of wild roses and freesia, punctuated with the spicy richness of ginger, cardamom and cinnamon. A warm base of grenadine, cedarwood and peach lingers on.

■ YVES SAINT LAURENT – PARIS
Classic floral
Eau de toilette, £35 for 50ml

Parisian elegance in a bottle. This classic fragrance is made to appeal to everyone and blends some 232 different notes. Light mimosa and hawthorn open the scent, unfolding into the main core of rose, iris and violet. A base of sandalwood, moss, amber and musk makes for lingering warmth.

CHYPRE/WOODY

BALENCIAGA – QUADRILLE
Classic mossy woody
Eau de toilette, £19.50 for 30ml
First brought out in 1955 and back by popular demand, this distinctive and elegant fragrance combines woody notes with delicious hints of citrus. A top note of bergamot leads into a heart of peach, rose and jasmine. However, the base notes of vetiver, oak moss, sandalwood and cedarwood are the most powerful.

CLARINS – EAU DYNAMISANTE
Light woody
Eau de toilette, £20 for 100ml; £28 for 200ml
A fragrance loved by both men and women alike, this is a light blend of 14 aromatherapeutic plant extracts and essential oils, expertly designed to lift the spirits. Citrus notes, including lemon and orange extract, mix with warmer notes of thyme, rosemary and ginger, plus a dash of patchouli to add depth.

CRABTREE & EVELYN – CAYMAN WINDS
Spicy woody
Eau de toilette, £17.50 for 100ml
A scent that captures the fresh island breezes of the West Indies. Fruity top notes of lemon, mandarin and bergamot caress a heart of sensual jasmine and ginger, before being followed by a base of sandalwood and orange blossom.

DIPTYQUE – PHILOSYKOS
Exotic woody
Eau de toilette, £28 for 50ml; £42.50 for 100ml
The founders of Diptyque wanted to capture the unique scent of a ripe Greek fig in this fresh and highly distinctive fragrance. Its notes use all parts of the fig tree – leaf, blossom, fruit, sap and resin – to compose a rich, multilayered aroma.

DOLCE & GABBANA – FEMININE
Floral woody
Eau de toilette, £48 for 100ml
Young, happy and assured, this is an energetic, flowery fragrance for everyday wear. Top notes of green pear, mimosa, wisteria and heliotrope skip towards a heart of jasmine and lily. Sweet, woody musk and sandalwood linger.

GIORGIO ARMANI – MANIA
Oriental woody
Eau de toilette, £37.50 for 50ml; £50 for 100ml
An enticingly exotic blend of spices and incense notes. The head notes are rich in citrus and pittospore, building to a spicy heart of saffron, clove, nutmeg and amber. Final richness is bestowed by a base of musk and Bourbon vanilla.

GRES – CABOCHARD
Oriental woody
Eau de parfum, £25 for 50ml
Inspired by a trip to India, this elegant, enigmatic perfume is a blend of floral and woody essences. Top notes of lichen and white flowers mingle with a core of tobacco, tangerine and leather, with base sandalwood and musk evoking rich Eastern spices.

GUCCI – GUCCI
Oriental woody
Eau de parfum, £26 for 30ml
Notes of citrus, cumin and thyme are fused with heliotrope and intertwined with orange blossom, orris, vanilla and deep musk, to create a complex, sexy fragrance that is essentially elegant, womanly and sophisticated – a truly great evening scent.

GUERLAIN – MITSOUKO
Fruity woody
Eau de parfum, £32 for 50ml
This classic perfume was inspired by a story of forbidden love: Mitsouko was married to a Japanese man, but fell hopelessly in love with a British soldier. Top notes of bergamot mingle with a rich heart of peach, rose and jasmine and are then emboldened by an earthy base of oak moss, spices and wood.

HERMES – CALECHE
Classic mossy woody
Eau de toilette, £24 for 30ml
A refined, flowery cypress scent, ideal for evening wear. Cheerful top notes of bergamot, orange and jasmine open and are enriched by rose, ylang ylang and iris middle notes. A base of musk intensifies the blend, making for a lingering aroma.

J. L0 – GLOW
Warm woody
Eau de toilette, £25 for 50ml spray; £35 for 100ml spray
Devised by the superstar herself to 'recreate the scent of bare, glowing skin that's been warmed by the heat of the body', this is a clean but sexy fragrance. Fresh top notes of neroli, orange blossom and pink grapefruit mingle with the seductive middles notes of rose, sandalwood and amber, with simple base notes of musk, jasmine and vanilla adding depth.

JO MALONE – FLEURS DE LA FORET
Classic mossy woody
Eau de toilette, £20 for 100ml
A delicate and elegant '1920s-style' scent, with a soft powdery finish. It begins with top notes of bergamot and rose, warming to a floral heart of iris, violet and jasmine, with a hint of clove and cumin. Tonka bean, oak moss and sandalwood combine for a sensuous base.

JOOP! – JOOP!
Rich oriental woody

Eau de toilette, £35 for 50ml

A fruity, modern scent with refreshing essence of bergamot, lemon and coriander to open, followed by notes of jasmine and lily of the valley at its heart. Cedarwood and sandalwood meanwhile provide warmth and depth at the base.

L'ARTISAN PARFUMEUR – VOLEUR DE ROSES
Warm woody

Eau de parfum, £39.50 for 50ml; £58 for 100ml

A soft and interesting scent enjoyed by both men and women, which blends fruit with wood. A fresh initial burst of bergamot, rose, apple and plum melts into a heart of patchouli leaves and sandalwood. The base, meanwhile, is comprised of sensual amber and musk.

LA PERLA – LA PERLA
Dry woody

Eau de parfum, £49 for 50ml

Indian carnation, freesia and jasmine grace this unique blend of herbs, spices and floral essences. Citrus notes, coriander and sandalwood are just some of the other highlights of this quietly seductive and sophisticated scent.

PALOMA PICASSO – PALOMA PICASSO
Floral woody

Eau de parfum, £39 for 50ml

Intensely passionate, this is not a perfume to wear when you are feeling meek and mild. Top notes of bergamot and citrus open the scent, warming to a heart of jasmine, hyacinth and ylang ylang. Finally, oak moss and sandalwood form the base of this sensual fragrance.

ROBERTO CAVALLI – ROBERTO CAVALLI
Sensual woody

Eau de parfum, £38 for 40ml

A cosmopolitan scent from this daring designer. The top notes include a fruity combination of tangerine, bergamot, magnolia and red apple, while the warm floral heart mixes freesia, wild orchid and cedarwood. A final richness is left on the skin – thanks to patchouli, Indian sandalwood, amber and musk.

SISLEY – EAU DE SOIR
Floral woody

Eau de parfum, £80 for 100ml

A refined, elegant perfume which is perfect for evenings. Citrus top notes of mandarin and grapefruit mingle with a sensuous floral and woody middle of jasmine, rose, lily of the valley, oak musk, pepper and clove. Amber and musk base notes add intensity and depth.

TRUSSARDI – TRUSSARDI DONNA
Fresh woody
Eau de toilette, £30 for 50ml
A timeless, feminine fragrance with a gorgeous mix of flowers, citrus notes and flashes of spice. Top notes include jasmine, mimosa and Bulgarian rose, and these lead into a rich middle of cypress. Musk, patchouli and Bourbon vetiver comprise the sensuous base.

VERSACE – VERSACE WOMAN
Floral woody
Eau de parfum, £35 for 50ml; £50 for 100ml
An extremely feminine perfume that is both seductive and elegant, it was created by blending notes of frangipani, bergamot and jasmine with the intense scent of padparadcha lotus and fruity hints of prune, raspberry, cedar, musk and amber.

FOUGERE

CALVIN KLEIN – BE
Fresh aromatic
Eau de toilette, £19.95 for 50ml; £28.75 for 100ml
Launched in 1996 as a unisex fragrance, this was accompanied by one of Klein's groundbreaking advertising campaigns featuring young, androgynous couples. A carefree scent that blends crispness with warmth, the top notes exude the tonic freshness of bergamot, juniper berry, mandarin and mint, while light spices, magnolia and succulent peach mix at the scent's core. Rich bottom notes of sandalwood and opopanax add a final musky flavour.

CREED – ROYAL WATER
Fresh green
Eau de parfum, £39.50 for 30ml
An uplifting and deliciously natural-smelling cocktail of citrus and spice that is said to have many celebrity followers. Its top note of hesperides blends seamlessly with the invigorating heart of basil, mint, juniper, pepper and cumin, and is rounded off with a satisfying base of musk and amber.

DIESEL – DIESEL ZERO PLUS FEMININE
Modern aromatic
Eau de toilette, £24.95 for 75ml
This unusual, youthful scent hits you with mouthwatering hints of cherry, coconut milk, strawberry and vanilla – an exotic, olfactory blend that perfectly complements the delicate middle of fruity florals and the base of exotic woods. It is a feminine and forward-looking fragrance, which comes encapsulated in a funky, futuristic red canister.

DIPTYQUE – EAU D'ELIDE
Classic aromatic
Eau de toilette, £28 for 50ml; £42.50 for 100ml

Warm and earthy, this sweet pastoral blend evokes the freshness of the aromatic shrubs of ancient Greece. Fruity top notes, including bitter orange blend with a crisp herbal centre of lavender, and rich musk and greenwood form the base notes.

ETRO – LEMON SORBET
Fresh aromatic
Eau de parfum, £48 for 100ml

A fresh, uplifting perfume, reminiscent of warm Mediterranean evenings and thus ideal for summer. A zingy lemon, orange peel and petitgrain opening carries you into a herbal middle note of lavender and rosemary. Sensual sandalwood and vetiver complete this delicious fragrance.

GUERLAIN – JICKY
Oriental aromatic
Eau de parfum, £32 for 30ml

Adored by Jackie Kennedy Onassis, this dry, feminine evening perfume was inspired by an ex-lover of the company's founder Aimé Guerlain. Invigorating top notes of bergmot and rosemary set the scene, and are followed by a sultry heart of rose, tonka bean, basil and fern. Rich woods and vanilla form a long-lasting base.

HUGO BOSS – HUGO DEEP RED
Rich aromatic
Eau de toilette, £29 for 50ml; £36 for 90ml

A distinctive, provocative scent to wear at night. Uplifting top notes of pear, cassis and blood orange blend into a floral core of pittosporum, hibiscus and ginger flower. A sensual mix of mysorwood, cedarwood, vanilla and musk add intensity.

ICEBERG – EFFUSION
Spicy aromatic
Eau de toilette, £25.00 for 75ml

A young, vibrant scent with top notes based on passionfruit, pink grapefruit and kiwi. The middle is an elegant floral bouquet of rose, jasmine and violet, circled by a warm blend of sensuous spices, such as nutmeg, clove and cardamom, while the soft, delicate base is of freesia petals and a woody blend of sandalwood and cedar.

PENHALIGON'S – ENGLISH FERN
Classic aromatic
Eau de parfum, £32 for 50ml; £44 for 100ml

A classic perfume that conjures up the crisp aroma of English woodland, its fresh, green aroma making it ideal for both men and women. Top notes of geranium and lavender provide a bracing opening; are followed by woody middle notes of oak moss and clover and rounded off by a warm base of patchouli and sandalwood.

ROGER & GALLET – EAU DE THE VERT
Fresh aromatic
Eau de toilette, £19.95 for 100ml
Delicate green tea makes this a revitalizing scent. Citrus top notes of mandarin, bergamot, grapefruit and lemon flow into a floral middle of orange blossom, freesia, jasmine and green tea. A base combines cedarwood, guayac wood and amber.

VIVIENNE WESTWOOD – LIBERTINE
Fruity aromatic
Eau de toilette, £25 for 30ml spray; £35 for 50ml spray
Westwood's latest fragrance is uplifting and sensuous. Grapefruit and pineapple top notes, set against invigorating bergamot, are succeeded by a middle of white florals, including lily of the valley, rose, honeysuckle and viburnum – the designer's favourite flower. Woody patchouli, oak moss and lusty amber provide base notes.

ORIENTAL

ALEXANDER MCQUEEN – KINGDOM
Rich oriental
Eau de parfum, £54 for 100ml
A fusion of the rare and exotic, this sensual fragrance is based around sandalwood. Top notes include bergamot, mandarin and neroli, intermingled with cumin, rose and jasmine petals. The base is formed of ginger, vanilla, myrrh and copah wood.

ALAIN BOUCHERON – BOUCHERON
Classic floral oriental
Eau de toilette, £40 for 50ml
This is a rich and voluptuous scent blending top notes of apricot, marigold and bitter orange, with middle notes of jasmine, orange blossom and broom and a semi-oriental base that includes sandalwood and tonka bean.

BURBERRY – TOUCH
Light oriental
Eau de parfum, £36 for 50ml spray
Headily intense Eastern vanilla and cedarwood complete a show opened by top notes that include tender fruits of dewberry, cassis and rosehip. Sensuality lies in the floral heart of tuberose, jasmine and Madonna lily, with peach and raspberry.

CACHAREL – CACHAREL
Fresh oriental
Eau de toilette, £25 for 50ml; £39 for 100ml
A delightful classic. Floral top notes of crushed hibiscus and roses blend with vanilla pods sparked with white pepper, tonka bean and benzoin. A whisper of ambergris at the base finishes this addictive fragrance.

CACHAREL – LOU LOU
Crisp floral oriental
Eau de parfum, £19.50 for 30ml
Cacharel regarded this perfume, combining 'tenderness and seduction', as best summed up by 1920s film star Louise Brooks. Using the Tahitian tiare flower with mimosa and heliotrope as middle notes and marigold, blackcurrant, sandalwood, incense and vanilla as other ingredients, it is a warm and provocative fragrance.

CARTIER – MUST DE CARTIER
Fresh oriental
Eau de parfum, £25 for 50ml
A long-lasting, seductive fragrance for true oriental devotees, this combines fresh, green mandarin and neroli with a classic bouquet of roses, daffodils and jasmine, before a final sultry note of musk and vetiver is introduced at the base.

CALVIN KLEIN – OBSESSION
Fresh oriental
Eau de parfum, £31 for 50 ml; £45 for 100ml
Florals and spices make this an intoxicating, warm and earthy perfume. It begins with top notes of mandarin, bergamot and subtle green nuances, mingling with middle notes of jasmine, orange blossom and exotic spices. Finally, bottom notes of amber, oak moss, incense and musk impart intensity.

CARON – NUIT DE NOEL
Classical woody oriental
Eau de parfum, £44 for 50ml
Created in 1922, this perfume captures the magic of the 1920s. It is a rich, festive fragrance with undertones of jasmine, rose, ylang ylang, vetiver, sandalwood and Mousse de Saxe, said to resemble the scent of a tiger's lair. Sensual and powerful.

CHANEL – COCO
Rich soft oriental
Eau de parfum, £48 for 50ml
Created in homage to Mademoiselle Chanel herself, Coco is a seductive, spicy fragrance, ideal for evening wear. The opening notes of angelica and orange blossom invite you into a rich, floral heart of Indian jasmine and Turkish rose. The woody base is deep and vibrant with final notes of vanilla and tonka bean.

CHRISTIAN DIOR – POISON
Rich fruity oriental
Eau de toilette, £24 for 30ml; £36.50 for 50ml
A mysterious and provocative scent – the 'power scent' of the 1980s – with enduring popularity. Orange and wild berries open this rich fragrance, followed by tuberose, coriander and pepper. Finally, honey, cinnamon and cistus labdanum give the long-lasting intensity for which it is renowned.

E. COUDRAY – AMBRE ET VANILLE
Classic oriental

Eau de parfum, £35 for 100ml

Edmund Coudray was court perfumier in the reign of Louis XVIII and founded his own fragrance shop in 1822. The ultimate in Parisian chic, this warming perfume begins with a swirl of bitter chocolate, sweet orange and ylang ylang, and then moves into a rich heart of cinnamon, iris and tonka bean, before finally softening to an intense finish of vanilla, amber and patchouli.

ESTEE LAUDER – INTUITION
Modern oriental

Eau de parfum, £36 for 50ml; £52 for 100ml

Traditionally fragrances have top, middle and base notes that unfold over time but, unusually, Intuition has three clearly distinct scents that release their aromas simultaneously. Amber, which provides a core of warmth and sensuality, is balanced on the one hand by a floral mix of rose, gardenia and freesia and, on the other, by a blend of sharp citrus.

ESTEE LAUDER – YOUTH-DEW
Rich oriental

Eau de parfum, £18.50 for 28ml; £26.50 for 65ml

Youth-Dew revolutionized the fragrance industry when it was created 50 years ago and it became one of the most popular and enduring perfumes of the twentieth century. The top note combines a bouquet of Bulgarian roses and jonquil with lavender, camomile and bergamot, for a delicate freshness. The heart is a blend of deeper floral notes, such as jasmine, ylang ylang and carnation, while exotic bottom notes of sandalwood, incense and musk supply warmth.

FENDI – FENDI
Rich woody oriental

Eau de toilette, £40 for 50ml

Created by the company founder's five daughters and their respective daughters, this fragrance combines patchouli and ylang ylang with jasmine and rose, sandalwood, musk, iris and amber, with dashes of spice. Leather, an appropriate addition but largely ignored as an ingredient since the 1920s and 1930s, was also included. The result is very Roman – flamboyant, sensual and enthusiastic.

GIORGIO ARMANI – SENSI
Floral oriental

Eau de toilette, £39 for 50ml; £56 for 100ml

The latest scent from fashion guru Giorgio Armani reflects his passion for the East. Opening with a refreshing top note of kaffir lime combined with cassis flower, it then blossoms with rich jasmine in the middle note. Palisander, an exotic wood with hints of vanilla and benzoin, is the dominant base note, and it creates a strong contrast with the fragrance's delicate floral core.

GIVENCHY – YSATIS
Fresh woody oriental
Eau de toilette, £34 for 50ml
Described by Givenchy as 'a perfume for a thousand women in one', this features
an intriguing combination of flowers, wood and spices. The rich mix of Egyptian
rose, iris, jasmine, ylang ylang and orange blossom reveals a base of sandalwood,
patchouli and musk. This is a lovely, heady and feminine fragrance.

GUERLAIN – SHALIMAR
Rich oriental
Eau de parfum, £28 for 50ml
Inspired by the love displayed by the Indian emperor who built the Taj Mahal for
his wife, this perfume has a fresh top note of bergamot and lemon, before leading
to a heart of rose and jasmine, with a hint of vanilla, and on to a powdery base
of incense and tonka bean.

JEAN-CHARLES BROSSEAU – OMBRE ROSE
Floral oriental
Eau de parfum, £40 for 50ml
This perfume has strong floral tones of rose, lily of the valley, iris and a surprising
glow of honey combined with the warmth of musk, sandalwood, vanilla and
peach. It is enigmatic, sensual and assured.

LANCOME – TRESOR
Crisp floral oriental
Eau de parfum, £30 for 50ml
Isabella Rossellini was chosen as the face to launch this perfume in 1990; her
feminine sensuality with a hint of mystery was deemed to sum up its character.
Top notes include white roses and lily of the valley while the fruity notes of apricot
liaise with a base that includes sandalwood and musk.

LAURA BIAGIOTTI – ROMA
Crisp oriental
Eau de toilette, £30 for 50ml
An alluring, dynamic and quintessentially Roman scent that combines cardamom
with bergamot and mint at the top, has a sweet heart of jasmine, rose, carnation and
lily of the valley, and patchouli, myrrh and oak moss as notable base notes.

LAURA MERCIER – L'HEURE MAGIQUE
Light oriental
Eau de toilette, £42 for 50ml
A clean but surprisingly rich fragrance. Top notes include cyclamen, pikake petals,
ylang ylang and a hint of violet – infused with the subtle scent of bergamot. White
roses, pink geraniums and osmanthus blossom make up the heart, while a base of
sandalwood, cashmere musk and amber give the fragrance its Eastern warmth.

LOLITA LEMPICKA –LOLITA LEMPICKA
Fresh oriental
Eau de parfum, £31 for 50 ml; £43 for 100ml

Created by the husband-and-wife team behind the French fashion label, this refreshing and yet intoxicating perfume combines aniseed and ivy top notes with a heady heart note of iris and violet flower. Finally, vetiver, vanilla and musk blend together to create spice and warmth. An enticing formula.

MICHAEL KORS – MICHAEL KORS
Light floral oriental
Eau de parfum, £49 for 50ml

Here is a perfume of contradictions: modern and classic, cool and warm. Michael Kors opens with top notes of freesia, incense and osmanthus, which warm to a heady heart of tuberose and peony. Finally, cashmere, woods and musk build a base of rich intensity.

MOSCHINO – MOSCHINO PARFUM
Rich oriental
Eau de toilette, £32 for 45ml

A sexy, spicy, provocative scent but one that is refined and lingering. Top notes of freesia and plum mingle with a rich heart of gardenia, clove and pepper. Base notes of exotic woods, amber and pepper give lasting depth.

OSCAR DE LA RENTA – VOLUPTE
Crisp floral oriental
Eau de toilette, £35 for 50ml

Rich, feminine and sensual, this is a heady mix of violet, jasmine and freesia that merges with the scents of ripe melon and mandarin combined with depths of incense, patchouli, sandalwood and musk.

ROCHAS – TOCADE
Floral oriental
Eau de toilette, £20 for 30ml

Launched in 1994, this classic floral oriental is a deeply sensual fragrance. Soft orange blossom top notes evolve into a blend of rose and vanilla, with amber at the base to create a vivacious and well-rounded composition.

SHISEIDO – FEMININITE DU BOIS
Classic woody oriental
Eau de parfum, £40 for 50ml

This sensual, feminine perfume, from the Japanese beauty and skincare company, is inspired by the cedarwood atlas tree, and the harmony and balance found in nature. It marries floral, fruity notes with hints of spice. The top, middle and base notes all contain different elements of cedarwood, with added spices, musk and amber providing warmth.

SPACE NK – WOMAN
Floral oriental
Eau de parfum, £48 for 60ml
Eau de toilette, £38 for 60ml
A modern yet elegant fragrance that is perfect for evening wear, this opens with the freshness of Italian bergamot, lemon and narcissus, a floral feel then further enriched with heart notes of jasmine, iris and lily. The base note rounds off the scent with cedarwood, amber and honey, for a sensual embrace.

THIERRY MUGLER – ANGEL
New oriental
Eau de parfum, £49 for 100ml
An innovative and distinctive perfume with plenty of impact. The light top note mixes fruits and honey, warming to a heart of vanilla, coumarine, chocolate and caramel. The culmination is a forceful woody base of patchouli.

VALENTINO – VERY VALENTINO
Floral oriental
Eau de toilette, £34 for 50ml
This is a refreshing oriental, oozing all the class and elegance that the designer's name represents. Citrus and floral top notes are fused with a heady heart of jasmine and rose. Final base notes of sandalwood, vanilla, amber and musk add harmony and richness.

YVES SAINT LAURENT – OPIUM
Classic oriental
Eau de toilette, £34.50 for 30ml; £44 for 50ml
A sophisticated, exotic blend of lush florals and rich spices, first introduced in 1977 to symbolize Yves Saint Laurent's fascination with the Orient. Tangerine, plum and cloves form the top notes, surrounding a heart of carnation, lily of the valley and rose, while myrrh, cedarwood and sandalwood conjure up lasting intensity at the base.

TIPS

- Woody/chypres, fougères and orientals are the classic choices for evening.
- Spray scent on your pulse points – behind the ears, the neck, the decollétage, the inner wrists and behind the knees.
- To give a delicate all-over body scent, spray the fragrance into the air and then walk through it.
- Take your time buying scent and do not buy on the first spray alone. The fragrance will need a few hours to develop on your individual skin.
- To keep fragrances fresh and lasting longer, store them in cool conditions away from direct sunlight.

CITRUS

ANNA SUI – SUI DREAMS
Floral citrus
Eau de toilette, £28 for 50ml; £36 for 75ml
This exhilaratingly fresh fragrance comes in a funky handbag-shaped bottle!
Top notes of bergamot, tangerine and peach fuse with a floral heart of freesia,
peony and rose. Finally, a base comprising notes of cedarwood, sandalwood
and vanilla completes this delicious scent.

AVEDA – CHAKRA 1 MOTIVATION SPIRIT
Floral citrus
Eau de toilette, £30 for 50ml
This fragrance is from a therapeutic range of seven chakra perfumes that contain
pure flower and plant extracts, developed in response to the ancient Ayurvedic
principle that says the body has seven energy centres or chakras that sometimes
become depleted. Different aromas are believed to help restore lost energy and
balance to each chakra. This particular combination of lemon, narcissus, olibanum
and vetiver is exhilarating and calming, to lift the spirits and boost confidence.

THE BODY SHOP – LEMON TEA
Crisp citrus
Eau de parfum, £18 for 50ml
Perfume oil, £12 for 20ml
An invigorating perfume that's full of life. Its top notes of Italian lemon
combine with crushed leaves and woody notes for a memorable impact.
The middle notes exude the crispness of lemon tree leaves and rose, along
with black Assam tea and green Chinese tea. Finally, the scent warms to woody
base notes of cedar and musk.

BULGARI – BULGARI EAU PARFUMEE
Fresh citrus
Eau de parfum, £44 for 75ml; £75 for 150ml
A fresh, delicate perfume inspired by the rituals of tea-making. It immediately
reveals citrus, jasmine and rose, before releasing the heart note of pure green tea.
Smoked wood, cardamom, pepper and coriander resonate with warmth and
spice at the base.

CHANEL – CRISTALLE
Crisp citrus
Eau de parfum, £48 for 50ml
Sparkling and youthful, this is an ideal perfume for sunny summer days.
A stimulating top note of Sicilian orange and peach introduces a green floral
heart of hyacinth and honeysuckle, enriched by jasmine and iris. Warmth and
woodiness are added by a base of vetiver and oak moss.

CHRISTIAN DIOR – DIORELLA
Floral citrus
Eau de toilette, £36.50 for 50ml; £52 for 100ml
A refreshing yet sophisticated fragrance with a rare combination of woody, fruity and citrus notes. Lemon and basil provide the uplifting top notes, while honeysuckle, peach and Moroccan jasmine form the heart. Finally, vetiver and oak moss comprise the base, providing an unforgettable finish.

ELIZABETH ARDEN – GREEN TEA
Fresh citrus
Eau de toilette, £18 for 50ml; £24 for 100ml
An uplifting and energizing scent based on deliciously refreshing green tea. Zingy top notes of lemon, rhubarb and peppermint open, and lead on to a heart of pure green tea, jasmine, celery seed and carnation, with an added hint of spice from caraway and fennel. Finally, musk and amber create a woody warmth.

GUERLAIN – PAMPLELUNE
Rich citrus
Eau de toilette, £23.50 for 75ml
An unusual combination of zesty fruits with florals and spices. Top notes of hesperides, Californian grapefruit and bergamot unfold into a heart of neroli, petitgrain and blackcurrant bud, warming to a patchouli and vanilla base.

HUGO BOSS – BOSS WOMAN
Floral citrus
Eau de parfum, £30 for 50ml; £37 for 90ml
A fruity, floral perfume, wonderful for daywear. It unfolds with the exotic scent of mandarin, mango and kumquat, which is built around a feminine centre of freesia, orris and passionflower. To give balance, a rich base of white cedar and sandalwood complete the fragrance.

MILLER HARRIS – CITRON CITRON
Fresh citrus
Eau de parfum, £52 for 50ml
A crisp and exotic perfume from London's Lyn Harris, one of the world's most innovative 'noses', this is a refreshing mix of Spanish orange, Sicilian lemon and Jamaican lime with cool notes of fresh mint leaves and sweet basil. The base is earthy – green moss, cedarwood and cardamom.

PACO RABANE – ULTRA VIOLET
Floral citrus
Eau de parfum, £20 for 30ml
This new fragrance is sure to quickly become a favourite as an everyday perfume. Zesty top notes of bergamot mix with a light floral heart of jasmine and violet. A touch of warmth is introduced with a base note of oak moss.

OZONIC

ADIDAS WOMAN – FITNESS EAU DE TOILETTE SPRAY
Crisp water
Eau de toilette, £7.50 for 20ml
A vibrant fragrance with all the freshness of crisp morning air. Ozonic top notes mingle with a light heart of citrus, while the base notes of sandalwood and amber leave a woody, musky finish. Ideal for everyday wear.

ARAMIS – NEW WEST FOR HER
Classic water
Eau de toilette, £29 for 30ml
A fresh, light blend of aquatic scents. The opening note is comprised of hyacinth and marigold, freshened with melon, mandarin and bergamot, plus herbal accents of basil, thyme and oregano. A heart of jasmine and rose is then spiced with clove and warmed with base notes of sandalwood, oak moss and patchouli.

CALVIN KLEIN – ESCAPE
Rich water
Eau de parfum, £37 for 50ml; £54 for 100ml
A truly romantic, fruity fragrance, light enough to wear during the day. Fresh, watery top notes of camomile, apple, lychee and mandarin blend with middle notes of jasmine, plum, clove and carnation. Finally, bottom notes of musk, sandalwood and vetiver unfold for lasting warmth.

LES EAUX DE CARON – EAU PURE
Oriental water
Eau de parfum, £44 for 50ml
A delightful marine blend, with a subtle spicy note, this scent can be worn by men and women alike. The fragrance opens with water fruits and passion fruit blossom, then warms to a fruity heart of bergamot and mandarin. A final flourish of warmth is added by rosewood, spice and cedar at the base.

DAVIDOFF – COOL WATER
Fresh water
Eau de toilette, £29.50 for 50ml; £40 for 100ml
A delicate but enduring fragrance that has become a modern classic. Fruity top notes of blackcurrant, pineapple and melon combine with a fresh floral blend of lotus blossom and water lily at the heart and a quirky touch of quince at the base.

ELIZABETH ARDEN – SUNFLOWERS
Floral water
Eau de toilette, £21 for 50ml; £30 for 100ml
A warm, bright scent with uplifting fruity overtones that make this a perfect summer scent; what is more, it can be worn safely in the sun. A fruity top note

of melon and peach mingles with rich floral notes of jasmine and tea rose at the heart, while deeper accents of sandalwood, moss and musk combine at the base for a soft but stylish finish.

ISSEY MIYAKE – L'EAU D'ISSEY
Crisp water
Eau de toilette, £37.50 for 50ml; £49.75 for 100ml
A truly modern scent, created to capture the 'essence of water'. Its light, feminine aroma makes it ideal as an everyday scent. Fresh notes of lotus, freesia and rosewater blend seamlessly into a floral heart of carnation, peony and lily. Finally, soft woods, tuberose and musk form a subtle base.

L'OCCITANE – FLEUR DE LOTUS
Crisp water
Eau de toilette, £25 for 100ml
A delightful flower water that is soft, but fragrant enough to last all day. Its opening notes blend white lily with marine elements, warming to a heart that is a bouquet of rose and jasmine. A woody base makes for a soft ending.

RALPH LAUREN – POLO SPORT WOMAN
Crisp floral water
Eau de toilette, £30.50 for 100ml
The ideal, all-over body fragrance with the light, clean aroma of soft floral and marines. Refreshing water mint, eucalyptus, melon and orange blossom open the scent, followed by a soft heart of lily, ylang ylang and freesia, tinged with the spiciness of nutmeg and ginger. Finally, a warm, woody base of bamboo, musk, oak and maple complete the blend.

TED BAKER – WOMAN
Fruity ozonic
Eau de parfum, £40 for 75ml
Eau de toilette, £30 for 75ml
A light, easy-to-wear fragrance that still manages to leave a lasting impression. The top notes are provided by a fruity combination of tangerine, apple and peach, while the heart is characterized by a softer, floral character with jasmine, freesia and ylang ylang, and a hint of spice from cinnamon. A subtle vanilla and musk undertone awaits at the base.

TOMMY HILFIGER – T GIRL
Floral ozonic
Eau de toilette, £29 for 50ml; £42 for 100ml
A sexy, young scent designed to invoke the crisp, clean breath of fresh air. It combines a top note of blackcurrant with a heart of tangerine, spearmint and violet for an invigorating, modern mood. The final base note is a rich blend of magnolia, cedar and sandalwood.

Sometimes beauty is skin deep; after all skin is the body's largest organ. While the appearance of skin is predominantly determined by genes, external and internal influences are important too, as skin will reflect your general wellbeing. Skin provides a protective barrier to factors like weather, UV rays and pollution, and acts as an inbuilt thermostat, helping to regulate temperature in accordance to the body's needs. But although it's amazingly adaptable, there are times when your skin needs a bit of extra help. For example, when you are not getting enough sleep or following a nutritious diet, you may suffer from a dull, spotty complexion. Other variables such as sunny holidays, cold weather and central heating can take their toll on the condition of your skin. The secret to combating such problems and maintaining a good complexion is to stick to a healthy, balanced diet, keep stress levels as low as possible and choose the right products to care for your skin.

Cleansing is fundamental to good skin, but too much can wash away the skin's natural oils and leave it irritated and dry. Soaps tend to be harsh, but soap-free cleansers are gentle and suitable for sensitive skin types. Cleansing milks and creams, based on oil emulsions and water, can be difficult to remove, but they are brilliant at dissolving dirt and make-up. Likewise, body washes should be chosen to meet your skin's needs, whether they are deep-cleansing or moisturizing.

The epidermis, or top layer of skin, continually creates new cells to replace the old ones, which flake off about once a month in a process called desquamation. Gentle exfoliation helps to remove these dead skin cells and can enhance a dull complexion, as well as diminish blocked pores and make skin better able to absorb moisturizer.

While moisturizing may be a necessary part of your routine, look at your skin before applying anything to it. Skin can change from season to season and through hormonal fluctuations so you may need to adapt your products for these times. If your skin is only dry around the cheek area, then apply moisturizer to just that area, or if your skin has a naturally moist appearance then you may not need any moisturizer at all. Many also contain sun protection, which dermatologists recommend to wear daily to protect against premature ageing and skin cancer.

Inevitably, skin will age, but thanks to phenomenal developments in dermatology, along with groundbreaking skincare products, you can help slow down this process. Many of the latest treatment creams and serums work to lift, brighten and improve the skin's retention of water, resulting in a more line-free, 'plumped-up' appearance. A beautiful, smooth complexion is obtainable if you take the time to understand your skin and its needs and choose the right products.

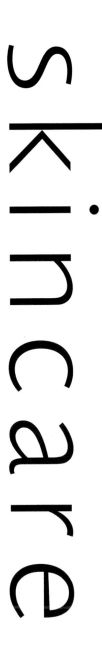

DAY MOISTURIZERS

■ AVEDA TOURMALINE CHARGED PROTECTION LOTION (SPF15)
Best for normal to oily skin

£32 for 75ml

Pure plant extracts including lemon, lime and lavender combine with the energizing mineral tourmaline, which is said to make plant ingredients more effective, in this light, oil-free lotion that enhances the skin's natural glow and helps to prevent sun damage. The healing power of tourmaline crystals works to harmonize and hydrate, so skin feels healthier as well as looking brighter.

■ AVENE SKIN RECOVERY CREAM
Best for very sensitive skin

£11.60 for 40ml

This light-as-air gel-cream contains 67 per cent water from the Avène thermal spring in France. It soothes irritated and even eczema-prone skin wonderfully, leaving skin feeling comfortable.

■ CHANEL DAILY PROTECTION LOTION (SPF25)
Best for daily sun protection

£12 for 30ml

This quickly absorbed oil-free lotion contains vitamin E and gives very high protection against UV rays. It helps firm and smooth skin, giving it a luminous glow.

■ CLARINS ENERGIZING MORNING CREAM (SPF15)
Best for all skin types, especially those with fine lines

£30 for 50ml

This superb anti-ageing cream is packed with vitamins and minerals, plus plant extracts and an anti-pollution complex. Its soft-focus pigments diminish the appearance of fine lines in bright daylight.

■ CLARINS HYDRATION-PLUS MOISTURE LOTION
Best for all skin types

£21.50 for 50ml

A great daily moisturizer, this safeguards skin against free-radical damage and UV rays, while boosting radiance. It not only has an immediate hydrating action but also increases skin's long-term ability to retain moisture. It contains honey, orange blossom and ginseng to soothe and tone skin.

■ CLINIQUE DRAMATICALLY DIFFERENT MOISTURIZING LOTION
Best for everyday use

£14 for 50ml

This 1968 classic is Clinique's bestselling product – a bottle is sold every two seconds. It has the same balance of oil and water as skin and is quickly absorbed to keep skin soft, supple and fresh. Also available in an oil-free formula.

CREME DE LA MER INTENSE MOISTURIZING CREAM
Best for dry or mature skin
£75 for 30ml

This deluxe wonder cream delivers visible anti-ageing results. Its sea kelp-based formula was originally developed by a NASA scientist to heal astronauts' burns, and it is also packed with vitamins and minerals, plus natural extracts, such as eucalyptus and sunflower oils. It is now available in a lotion for normal skin.

DERMALOGICA ACTIVE MOIST (SPF15)
Best for oily skin
£20.75 for 52ml

A lightweight, oil-free moisturizer, this contains active ingredients such as cucumber, burdock, sage and mallow. Its acid-balanced formula and softening emollients thoroughly moisturize while natural astringents guard against excess oiliness. It comes with a built-in sunscreen to help guard against environmental irritants and sun damage.

ESTEE LAUDER IDEALIST SKIN REFINISHER
Best for perfecting skin tone
£43 for 50ml

Idealist's exclusive non-acid formula speeds up the skin's shedding cycle, reducing fine lines and open pores, evening skin tone and leaving skin noticeably smoother. Anti-ageing ingredients include whey protein to help plump up skin, while a megadose of antioxidant vitamins fights free radicals.

ESTEE LAUDER RE-NUTRIV ULTIMATE LIFTING CREME
Best for mature skin
£150 for 50ml

Crushed South Sea pearls, white birch and kava kava are just three of the 50 exotic ingredients combined in this 'platinum'-quality cream that improves skin tone quickly and gives gentle luminosity. Its firming properties make it ideal for mature skin.

TIPS

- Don't apply cream to damp skin – it doesn't help 'trap' moisture but will simply dilute the product, making it less effective.
- Only use a five-pence-size amount of cream – any more can overload skin.
- For those with combination skin, choose a moisturizer that contains AHAs, which can help normalize both oily and dry areas.
- If you have dry skin, you may prefer to use a moisturizer on top of a firming treatment or serum; other skin types may benefit from using just one cream.
- Rather than using a separate sun block, in addition to a moisturizer, choose a day cream that contains an SPF of at least 15 to protect from UV damage.

■ GATINEAU LASER COMFORT DAY CREAM
Best for dry skin

£41.50 for 50ml

The marine ingredients in this rich cream soothe and protect skin, as 'energizing spheres' and 'light captors' reinforce the benefits of light and provide more energy for cell turnover and function. It's easily absorbed, giving soft, supple skin.

■ GIVENCHY NO SURGETICS
Best for firmer-looking skin

£40 for 50ml

This state-of-the-art moisturizer has a light texture that leaves skin ultra-smooth and 'lifted'. It contains an ingredient to help relax frown lines and in trials has been found to reduce wrinkles by 30 per cent after just four weeks' use.

■ GUERLAIN ISSIMA SUBSTANTIFIC HIGH-DENSITY NOURISHING DAY CREAM (SPF10)
Best for very dry skin

£66 for 50ml

A super-rich moisturizer that protects against cold and harsh winds – ideal for extra-dry skin that needs nourishing, but can double as a neck cream. Try Guerlain Happylogy Day Crème (£32.50 for 30ml), too, which is designed to increase the activity of cells responsible for fighting wrinkles.

■ JING JANG CREME
Best healing cream

£15 for 28.35g

Packed full of organic ingredients such as calendula flower, olive oil, sweet almond oil, beeswax and vitamin E, this gentle multipurpose cream is effective for everything from sunburn and minor abrasions to razor burn and bruises. It can also be used to give skin a subtle sheen. All-natural ingredients and its versatility of use make it a cult favourite.

■ KIEHL'S ULTRA FACIAL MOISTURIZER (SPF15)
Best for normal to dry skin

£27.70 for 100ml

This easily absorbed, conditioning formula, recommended by dermatologists and make-up artists, contains skin-compatible oils derived from avocado, apricot kernel, sweet almond and olives. The tinted version contains a sunscreen.

■ LANCOME ABSOLUE REPLENISHING CREAM (SPF15)
Best for brightening mature skin

£72.50 for 50ml

France's number one anti-ageing cream, Absolue is packed with natural ingredients such as sea kelp and wild yam. It is superb for mature skin (40 plus) because it brightens and firms the skin and reduces signs of sun damage.

■ LA PRAIRIE CELLULAR TIME-RELEASE INTENSIVE MOISTURIZER (SPF15)
Best preventative moisturizer
£85 for 30ml

This luxurious yet lightweight formula keeps skin moisturized for 16 hours, while improving elasticity. Based on an exclusive 'cellular' formula, designed to replenish the skin's natural vitamins and minerals, it's pricey but devotees say it's worth it.

■ L'OCCITANE IMMORTELLE PRECIOUS CREAM
Best botanical-based anti-wrinkle moisturizer
£29 for 50ml

Named after its key ingredient, the immortelle plant, which has been found to be exceptionally effective in the fight against free radicals and wrinkles, this moisturizer contains essential oil extracted from the flower. It also includes vitamins A and E to maximize the results. Used morning and evening, it helps to soften and reinvigorate tired skin.

■ NEAL'S YARD REMEDIES FRANKINCENSE NOURISHING CREAM
Best natural moisturizer
£10.25 for 40g

A rich cream with natural ingredients such as age-defying frankincense and myrrh, plus nourishing oils of almond, apricot kernel, jojoba and wheatgerm, this moisturizes dry skin deeply and treats fine lines. It can be used as a night cream in addition to a day make-up base.

■ NIVEA VISAGE Q10 PLUS ANTI-WRINKLE REPAIR CREAM
Best budget moisturizer for mature skin
£9.45 for 50ml

Co-enzyme Q10 is a natural antioxidant found in every cell of the body. This reasonably priced cream diminishes fine lines and smooths skin, and is available in both a day and a night formula.

■ OLAY TOTAL EFFECTS 7X DAY CREAM (SPF15)
Best budget moisturizer with SPF
£18.50 for 100ml

Skin-enhancing panthenol, as well as vitamins E and C, green tea extracts, zinc, magnesium and titanium dioxide combine to deliver a moisturizer that is both anti-ageing and protective.

■ ORIGINS MAKE A DIFFERENCE SKIN REJUVENATING TREATMENT
Best for sun-damaged skin
£25 for 50ml

Ideal for those concerned about the risks of sun exposure, this lightweight cream, with a refreshing scent of lemon, orange and bergamot, is full of botanical extracts that repair and moisturize deep in the dermis. It gives an instant glow to all skins.

■ PHILOSOPHY HOPE IN A JAR
Best for skin smoothing
£30 for 56.7g

A favourite with celebrities and make-up artists, this contains betaglucan, a powerful antioxidant, and lactic acid to smooth skin and bestow a healthy, rosy glow. Now also available is Hope in a Jar for Dry Skin, which contains protective vitamins A and F as well as other effective antioxidants, and is great for harsh weather conditions.

■ PRESCRIPTIVES MAGIC INVISIBLE LINE SMOOTHER
Best gel for filling in lines
£27 for 15ml

An innovative, waxy, silicon-based gel, this literally fills in wrinkles, sitting in lines and plumping up the skin. It works to fill in cracks, but also has special 'optical diffusers' that bounce back light for a soft-focus effect. Apply the gel carefully before moisturizer and foundation.

■ SHISEIDO FUTURE SOLUTION TOTAL REVITALIZING CREAM
Best for anti-ageing
£130 for 50ml

It took Shiseido's scientists nine years of research to perfect this effective anti-ageing cream. Delicately scented with white lotus and 'space' rose, this luxurious emulsion noticeably reduces the appearance of fine lines and wrinkles while firming the skin. The light gel formula melts into the skin, leaving it silky and soft. In tests over 80 per cent of users reported having firmer skin after using this product for a month.

■ SISLEY EMULSION ECOLOGIQUE
Best for combating free radicals
£75 for 125ml

This is a multivitamin- and mineral-rich light emulsion that promotes collagen production with essential oils of marine and plant extracts, as well as ginseng, rosemary and hops. It provides good defence against pollution and climate changes, and leaves skin feeling refreshed and toned. It can be used alone as a moisturizer or under another one if your skin is particularly dry. It's ideal for sensitive skin that is in need of a nutrient boost.

■ SJAL CELA INTUITIF CREAM
Best for renewing oily skin
£165 for 59ml

This lightweight day cream is designed to promote cellular renewal while gently tightening pores. Ingredients include echinacea and Sjal's rejuva-complex to help to diminish the appearance of wrinkles, algaes and pearl powder to even pigmentation and to moisturize, plus green tea and vitamins A, C and E to protect against free radicals.

NIGHT TREATMENTS

■ALMAY KINETIN REPAIR AND REJUVENATE NIGHT CONCENTRATE
Best for repairing damage

£18.95 for 40ml

Kinetin is a stable antioxidant found in both green leafy plants and human DNA; it is also the active ingredient of this cream, which helps to delay the onset of ageing in skin cells. It is especially suitable for sensitive skin and also an effective treatment for uneven pigmentation and dry, or rough, patches.

■CAUDALIE VINOLIFT TOTAL NIGHT CARE
Best antioxidant cream

£32 for 30ml

Beloved of actress Jennifer Aniston, this cult product contains antioxidants found in grape vines that smooth away signs of stress and ageing while you sleep.

■ CHRISTIAN DIOR CAPTURE R60/80 NUIT – INTENSE WRINKLE NIGHT FLUID
Best for anti-ageing

£36 for 30ml

Retinol and Dior's unique CURE complex form a deeply penetrating, intense night cream designed to reinforce skin elasticity and smoothness and decrease the depth – and therefore appearance – of wrinkles.

■ CLINIQUE REPAIRWEAR INTENSIVE NIGHT CREAM
Best for energizing

£45 for 50ml

This luxurious cream sinks easily into the skin. It contains a new complex called Vital Fuel, which enhances the skin's natural capability to produce energy. Having received moisture throughout the night, skin looks dewy and re-energized by dawn.

■ GUERLAIN MIDNIGHT SECRET
Best for overnight rejuvenation

£49.50 for 30ml

This miracle cream beloved of supermodels contains active ingredients that stimulate the circulation and increase oxygen into the skin while you sleep. The fine, silky emulsion glides on smoothly, and its unique blend of pure gold and marine algae will help your skin to recuperate rapidly after a big night out!

■ LANCOME PRIMORDIALE INTENSE NUIT
Best for radiance

£41.50 for 50ml

A rich moisturizer containing vitamin A and antioxidants, this works to repair daytime damage and keep the first signs of ageing at bay. Microcapsules release these nutrients throughout the night so that skin looks radiant next morning.

■ ORIGINS NIGHT-A-MINS
Best natural ingredient-based revitalizer

£22.50 for 50ml

Available in a cream or gel, this is packed with invigorating ingredients, including vitamin A to increase skin's strength and firmness, vitamin B to recharge moisture reserves, and folic acid to enhance skin renewal. It also has a relaxing scent to help you drift off to sleep, allowing your skin to regenerate to the maximum overnight.

SERUMS

■ AVEDA BIO-MOLECULAR PERFECTING FLUID
Best for smoothing

£28 for 30ml

This botanical skin serum is formulated to incorporate natural antioxidants, as well as AHAs and BHAs to remove dead skin cells and unclog pores. If you use this regularly before your moisturizer, you should see a reduction of lines and age spots in a matter of weeks. It leaves skin feeling healthier, softer and firmer.

■ BIOTHERM SOURCE THERAPIE
Best for revitalizing stressed skin

New release, price TBC

The silicones in this revitalizing serum will help boost the penetration and effectiveness of your usual moisturizer, making your face feel silky to the touch.

■ CHANEL HYDRA SERUM VITAMIN MOISTURE BOOST
Best for dehydrated skin

£31 for 30ml

Use this alone on dry skin or blend it with your favourite moisturizer. It is ideal for dehydrated winter skin or on long-haul flights.

■ CLARINS TOTAL DOUBLE SERUM
Best for dry and mature skins

£42 for 15ml

The latest version of this ever-popular product contains extra-firming ingredients, making it a great product for mature skin. It will also soothe skin that has been dried out by harsh winter conditions.

■ DOCTOR'S DERMATOLOGIC FORMULA WRINKLE RELAX (FAUX-TOX)
Best for line reduction

£65 for 15ml

A needle-free alternative to the now-fashionable Botox injections, this serum contains copper peptides that aim to temporarily freeze the muscles, lessening the depth and overall appearance of lines. It promises a visible reduction in lines after 45 days or sooner.

ESTEE LAUDER ADVANCED NIGHT REPAIR
Best for overall skin damage
£43 for 50ml
Packed full of antioxidant ingredients, this serum repairs by night and protects by day, helping to eliminate fine lines and giving skin a fresh, smoother look. It includes anti-inflammatory ingredients such as cola nut extract to help guard against environmental irritation and general skin damage.

GATINEAU DEFY LIFT 3D REDEFINING SERUM
Best for over-35s
£25 for 25ml
A complexion-lifting cocktail of soya peptides, almond proteins, and vitamins A and F, this should be applied twice a day for a month for a sensational skin boost.

JURLIQUE HERBAL EXTRACT RECOVERY GEL
Best natural serum for all skin types
£40.45 for 30ml
Rich in antioxidants and herbal extracts from plants including roses, daisies, marshmallow and camomile, this organic gel also includes extracts from green tea, grapeseed and turmeric to protect against cell damage and free radicals. Use under moisturizer when skin is dry or mature, or alone if normal to oily.

LA PRAIRIE CELLULAR RETEXTURIZING BOOSTER
Best for rapid refinement
£95 for 15ml
This cool, gel-like serum is non-irritating because it is based on aloe vera. Rapidly retexturizing the skin for a smoother appearance, it contains AHAs and BHAs to reduce fine lines and discoloration and La Prairie's exclusive cellular complex to nourish the skin. Use two drops only before moisturizing.

LA PRAIRIE SWISS CELLULAR SERUMS
Best luxury serum
£95 for 30ml
There are six advanced formulas in this range to treat every skin type and problem. Designed to hydrate, desensitize, retexturize, illuminate, reduce wrinkles or control oil, they take needy skin to nirvana.

LIZ EARLE SMOOTHING LINE SERUM
Best for lines around the eyes, lips and forehead
£10.50 for 10ml
Specially formulated as an intensive overnight treatment, this easily absorbed, light-textured serum treats fine lines on the face, including any around the lip and eye areas. Ingredients include echinacea to strengthen the skin, grapeseed extract to help protect against free radical damage, and natural-source vitamin E to help discourage signs of ageing.

■ PRADA REVIVING BIO-FIRM CONCENTRATE
Best for restoring skin
£92 for 15 x 10ml

The blend of collagen-making and skin-firming ingredients in this product includes retinol and vitamins C and E, along with essential fatty acids such as sunflower and meadow flower seed oils. This lightweight conditioning oil helps to reduce lines and firm and plump up the skin, leaving it looking more youthful and glowing.

■ SISLEY SISLEYA ELIXIR
Best for combating stress and fatigue
£180 for 4 x 5ml

A once-a-month treatment of four ampoules designed to give the face a total overhaul. It improves skin condition and reduces signs of stress and fatigue. Rich botanicals help to improve the appearance of wrinkles, leaving the overall texture of skin dramatically smoother.

■ THALGO L'ELIXIR
Best for smoothing and refining damaged skin
£120 for 4 x 10ml

Natural algae extracts form the foundation of this four-week serum course, which is formulated to give a youthful glow and new smoothness to skin in need of repair. Lost moisture is replenished, lines smoothed and skin is given additional protection from future environmental damage.

■ ZIRH SKIN NUTRITION CORRECT
Best for combating environmental damage
£22 for 50ml

Packed with natural oils and botanicals, this moisturizing skin serum helps to smooth out roughness, guard against irritation and keep skin soft and supple. Its multivitamins also help to shield the skin from free radicals and environmental damage. A favourite among New York celebrities, it's designed to cater for guys as well as girls, whatever the skin type.

MOISTURIZING FACIAL MASKS

■ AVON SUPER HYDRATING COOLING MASK
Best budget pick-me-up
£6 for 75ml

A great quick-fix when you're in a hurry, this mask takes effect in only a matter of seconds, and yet leaves skin feeling moisturized, fresh and tingly. It contains antioxidants that brighten the skin and help to combat fine lines. Simply massage into clean, dry skin and rinse thoroughly for firmer, more supple skin in an instant.

■ CHRISTIAN DIOR MASQUE COCOON
Best for tired, parched skin
£19.50 for 50ml
Intriguingly, this mask changes colour from pink to violet as it works. It is lightly scented with sage, lemon and mandarin, and soothing botanicals, including rose distillate, mallow extract and hibiscus, comprise its moisturizing content. As it works it clears dead cells, transforming a tired, parched complexion into a revived, luminous one.

■ DERMALOGICA INTENSIVE MOISTURE MASK
Best for dry skin
£28.80 for 74ml
This rich, creamy-textured mask contains natural honey and gingko biloba to revitalize dull skin. When first applied it can feel slightly tight and tingly, but it leaves dry skin newly hydrated, smooth and soft. For best results use once a week after exfoliating.

■ ESTEE LAUDER SO MOIST DEEP HYDRATING MASK
Best for deep hydration
£20 for 75ml
Fossilized mineral water containing copper, potassium, selenium and zinc, boosts the strength of the moisturizing benefits of this effective hydrating mask. Other ingredients include sweet almond and rice bran oils that keep skin soft and smooth. Great for when the seasons are changing, if you are travelling or are feeling stressed, or if you work in an air-conditioned office.

■ GUERLAIN ISSIMA INVIGORATING MOISTURIZING MASK
Best for nourishing
£24 for 75ml
Containing mallow, renowned for its moisturizing properties, this is a deep-moisturizing and refreshing mask especially good for dry or tired skin. It boasts Calmitine-S, a complex of soothing, protective active ingredients that combats potential irritants, guards against pollution and helps to retard the ageing process.

■ LA PRAIRIE CELLULAR MOISTURE MASK
Best for skin exposed to harsh external factors
£63 for 30ml
Deeply nourishing, this deep-repairing mask is ideal for use during the harsh winter months or after sun exposure.

■ LANCOME HYDRA INTENSE
Best gel hydrator
£22 for 100ml
This hydrating gel mask contains an extract of the imperata cylindrica plant, which is a natural water captor, helping to hold in moisture. It leaves skin soft and toned.

■ LIZ EARLE INTENSIVE NOURISHING TREATMENT
Best for all skin types

£8.50 for 50ml

This super-rich mask is crammed with skin-saving nutrients, including borage oil, shea butter, comfrey extract and soothing St John's wort. Delicately fragranced with rose geranium, this is suitable for all skin types, including sensitive skins. For best results, remove with the muslin washcloth included, soaked in hot water.

■ NIVEA VISAGE SOFT CALMING MASK
Best budget soothing mask

£1.25 for 15ml

This creamy mask relaxes stressed skin and restores its natural moisture balance. It contains aloe vera and camomile to help calm irritation and replace lost moisture so skin is left supple and soft.

■ PHILOSOPHY HOPE IN A JAR SUPER HYDRATING MASK
Best for quick hydration

£22 for 56.7g

Superb for stressed-out skin that needs instant rehydration, this mask plumps and smooths the skin. Formulated with a lightweight emulsion texture, it contains vitamin E (encapsulated in jojoba) to soothe, green tea extract to reduce puffiness and cucumber extract to calm the skin. Best used before bed or ten minutes before applying make-up.

■ SHISEIDO THE SKIN CARE MOISTURE RELAXING MASK
Best for revitalizing

£28 for 50ml

Ingredients include glycerine, thyme and tea rose extracts, as well as Shiseido's unique phyto-vitalizing factor. For best results try the face massage techniques detailed in the accompanying leaflet.

■ SISLEY EXPRESS FLOWER GEL MASK
Best for improved skin's surface tone

£43 for 60ml

This beautifully scented botanical mask leaves skin deeply hydrated and toned after just three minutes. Ingredients include organically grown sesame for a deep-penetrating moisture boost and iris and lily for a refreshing scent. Formulated for all skin types, it is especially good if skin has become dull and tired.

■ SK-II FACIAL TREATMENT MASK
Best radiance enhancer

£45 for 6 sachets

SK-II's unique magic ingredient is pitera, an extract from the fermentation process of the Japanese drink sake. Apparently it boosts radiance and moisture levels, leaving skin glowing with health.

CLEANSING FACIAL MASKS

■ AVEDA DEEP CLEANSING HERBAL CLAY MASQUE
Best fast-acting mask
£20 for 127g

This cool, aromatic mask is formulated with a unique mix of three clays that deep-cleanse and refresh the skin. These combine with moisturizing vitamin E, coconut and herbal essences, plus echinacea, red clover and hyssop to help purify and tone. The mask draws out impurities and gives skin a boost in just three minutes.

■ AVON PORE-FECTION CLEANSING MASK
Best budget buy for drawing out impurities
£4 for 75ml

A hardworking, three-in-one treatment that peels away dirt and oil while gently exfoliating dry, flaky skin. Suitable for normal/oily skin, it visibly reduces enlarged pores. Use two or three times a week for best results.

■ DEAD SEA SPA MAGIC ALGIMUD ACTIVE SEAWEED MASK
Best for travel
£2.99 for 25g

These sachets, ideal when you are travelling light, contain a powder that is made of pure Dead Sea mud mixed with crushed algae. It detoxifies and brightens tired skin, improves circulation, re-hydrates, soothes and cools – an ideal pick-me-up for you and your skin after a long journey.

■ DR HAUSCHKA REJUVENATING MASK
Best for a healthy glow
£22 for 30ml

An intensive mask that improves the condition of all skin types, this reduces the appearance of large pores while adding much-needed vitality to dry skin. It also acts as a gentle exfoliant to brighten pale or dull skin.

TIPS

- To tackle stubborn blackheads apply a mask that contains clay. It will help absorb impurities and soften the skin, making extraction easier.
- After a day in the sun, apply a calming mask to pump some moisture back into dehydrated pores and soothe soreness.
- Avoid exfoliating masks if you have sensitive skin, as they can be abrasive.
- If too many late nights have left skin tired and lifeless, choose a revitalizing mask to tighten pores, boost circulation and leave skin radiant.
- If skin is tired, stressed or parched, treat it with care. Do not over cleanse or exfoliate, instead apply a deeply moisturizing, vitamin-packed mask that will rejuvenate and repair the skin.

■ ELEMIS FRUIT ACTIVE REJUVENATING MASK
Best for refining skin
£21.50 for 75ml
A cleansing and refining mask, this incorporates strawberry and kiwi fruit extracts in a clay base, and contains macadamia nut oil to help eliminate toxins, and shea butter for natural moisture. A brilliant treatment for lacklustre or grey-looking skin.

■ FRESH ROSE FACE MASK
Best for mature skin
£ 36.50 for 100ml
This indulgent treatment will leave even delicate skin rejuvenated and relaxed. It is infused with crushed rose petals and has a delicate texture that just melts into the skin. Your face is left deeply hydrated and toned.

■ ORIGINS OUT OF TROUBLE MASK
Best for blemish-prone skin
£15 for 100ml
The ultimate rescue remedy for problem skin, this mask contains zinc oxide and sulphur to absorb excess oil and protect, camphor to soothe overreactive skin, plus salicylic acid to slough away dead skin cells. It refines the skin's texture, calms redness and reduces oil and shine.

EYE CREAMS

■ AVEDA TOURMALINE CHARGED EYE CREAM
Best for fine lines
£25 for 15ml
This botanical cream diminishes lines while the energizing mineral tourmaline leaves skin feeling fresh and supple. Other ingredients include refreshing lime and organic petitgrain essential oils and the antioxidant lycopene, a tomato extract that helps to protect the delicate eye area and also reduces puffiness.

■ THE BODY SHOP CHAMOMILE MOISTURIZING EYE SUPPLEMENT
Best budget buy for sensitive skin
£7.50 for 15ml
A soft, gel-like lotion with soothing camomile, this moisturizes the delicate skin around the eye without causing sensitivity.

■ CHRISTIAN DIOR CAPTURE R60/80 YEUX WRINKLE EYE CREAM
Best anti-wrinkle treatment for the eye area
£29 for 50ml
This is a hardworking cream that actively combats daily skin stressors such as pollution, cigarette smoke and fatigue using high-performance active ingredients such as retinol and antioxidants.

CLARINS EYE CONTOUR GEL

Best for puffiness

£18.50 for 20ml

A gentle eye gel containing butcher's broom and wild rose, this is brilliant for reducing puffiness and dark circles.It's ultralight and non-oily, so it won't overmoisturize the delicate eye area.

CLE DE PEAU BEAUTE EYE CREAM

Best for protection

£75 for 15ml

This excellent but expensive Japanese eye cream is infused with retinol to diminish fine lines. ('Clé de peau' is French meaning 'key to the skin'). It also contains UV filters to help protect the eye area from sun damage.

CLINIQUE ALL ABOUT EYES

Best for dark circles

£20 for 15ml

This lightweight gel has an instantly cooling effect and diminishes puffy eyes, dark circles and fine lines. The matt formula helps to keep make-up in place and protects skin against environmental damage.

DR HAUSCHKA EYE SOLACE

Best natural eye cream for sensitive eyes

£16 for 10 x 5ml

Pure plant ingredients, such as eyebright, fennel extract and rose essential oil, in this cooling lotion leave the eye area soothed and refreshed. This is wonderful for restoring tired, red eyes at the end of a hard day.

E'SPA SOOTHING EYE LOTION

Best for soothing

£12.50 for 50ml

Cucumber extract and cornflower make this an ideal soother for tired, puffy eyes.

GARNIER SYNERGIE STOP ANTI-AGEING EYE CONTOUR CREAM

Best budget buy for anti-ageing cream

£7.99 for 15ml

The latest technology, combining pure retinol and vitamin C, is hard at work in this cream, reducing the appearance of fine lines and encouraging cell renewal.

GUERLAIN ISSIMA EYE MYTHIC

Best for relaxing and restoring eye area

£26 for 15ml

A blend of plant-based ingredients, including beech bud, works to soothe and decongest the eye area, while oubaka extract refreshes it. The cream also helps to reduce puffiness and fade dark circles.

■ LANCOME ANTI-WRINKLE AND FIRMING EYE TREATMENT
Best for anti-ageing

£31.50 for 15ml

Although slightly oily in texture, this eye cream is quickly absorbed and feels cool and refreshing. It leaves skin around the eye area feeling noticeably more taut.

■ L'OREAL PLENITUDE HYDRAFRESH EYES
Best for refreshing tired eyes

£6.99 for 15ml

Low-priced yet extremely effective, this hydrating gel-cream, enriched with vitamins, is a favourite of dermatologists and make-up artists.

■ MARIO BADESCU CERAMIDE HERBAL EYE CREAM
Best for firming

£15.90 for 14g

A unique soothing and moisturizing formula that eases away fine lines caused by dryness, stress and harsh weather conditions. It also contains natural AHAs to encourage skin renewal. Gentle enough to be used by all skin types.

■ NIVEA VISAGE Q1O PLUS
Best budget buy, multifunctional eye cream

£9.45 for 15ml

This great-value eye cream is ophthalmologically tested and fragrance-free.Its active ingredient is co-enzyme Q10, which occurs naturally in every cell and stimulates the skin's regenerative and protective functions.

■ ORLANE B21 BIO-ENERGIC ABSOLUTE SKIN RECOVERY CONCENTRATE EMERGENCY CARE FOR EYES
Best for all-purpose eye care

£40 for 15ml

Ginseng extract and glucose reduce the appearance of fine lines, dark circles and puffiness in this impressively effective product.

■ OLE HENRIKSEN ULTIMATE LIFT EYE GEL
Best for soothing overnight

£31 for 28g

This star-endorsed prescription for puffy and bleary eyes gives sparkling results overnight, thanks to herbs and botanical agents.

■ PRESCRIPTIVES SUPER LINE PREVENTOR PLUS EYE CARE
Best for diminishing the appearance of fine lines

£30 for 15ml

The secret here is a combination of an exclusive skin recharging complex to speed up the repair process and magnolia to eliminate dark circles and reduce puffiness. The soothing gel formula also has a cooling effect on the skin.

■ **SHISEIDO BENEFIANCE REVITALIZING EYE CREAM**

Best for sensitive eyes

£32.50 for 15ml

This rich but gentle eye cream is extremely soothing and can be applied all over the eye area without fear of causing irritation. LAG Revitalizer and extract of ginseng encourage the normalization of plasmin in the skin to promote hydration and radiance while simultaneously diminishing the appearance of fine lines.

■ **YVES SAINT LAURENT SMOOTHING EYE CONTOUR GEL**

Best for invigorating the eye area

£28 for 15ml

Filled with high-tech ingredients, this gel is fantastic for keeping fine lines at bay. Apply it in the morning to refresh the eye area – your make-up will last longer too.

NECK CREAMS

■ **CHANEL PRECISION ULTRA-CORRECTION ANTI-WRINKLE RESTRUCTURING LOTION FOR FACE AND NECK (SPF 15)**

Best for mature skin

£42 for 50ml

This rich lotion contains shea butter, liquorice, canola oil, vitamin E and glutamic acid to boost skin's self-defence mechanism. Regular use will get the best results.

■ **CLARINS EXTRA FIRMING NECK CREAM**

Best for firming

£32.50 for 50ml

The antioxidant vitamin E, plus marine extracts, ginseng, mallow, olive extract and honey ensure that this lightly scented formula produces remarkable results. Its lightweight texture means that it can be used in the morning and/or before bed at night.

■ **DECLEOR VITAROMA LIFT TOTAL RE-SCULPTING CREAM FOR THE FACE AND NECK**

Best cream for face and neck

£54.50 for 50ml

A light yet luxurious cream-gel that sinks in instantly and 'tightens' looseness on the neck. The Vitaroma range combines pure botanical extracts with a unique phyto-hormone complex and essential oils, including those of lemongrass and iris.

■ **ELEMIS VITAL NECK FIRMING CREAM**

Best for deep nourishment

£26.50 for 30ml

This aromatherapeutic blend of royal jelly, propolis and jojoba, all rich in amino acids, minerals and vitamin B complex, retains moisture levels and nourishes skin.

■ ESTEE LAUDER RE-NUTRIV INTENSIVE LIFTING CREAM FOR THROAT AND DECOLLETAGE

Best for diminishing pigmentation

£70 for 50ml

This rich cream includes extract of green tea to reduce lines and the pigmentation caused by sun damage. AHAs gently refine the skin and smooth fine lines while helping to prevent the breakdown of collagen.

■ JURLIQUE NECK SERUM

Best natural neck serum

£47.25 for 30ml

Like all Jurlique products, this firming serum is formulated with entirely natural and organic ingredients. These include oils of frankincense and myrrh, for their revitalizing properties, ginkgo and soy bean extracts for protecting against cell damage and ageing, and seaweed extract to help reduce moisture loss.

■ LANCASTER SURACTIF NECK AND DECOLLETE TREATMENT

Best for softening

£42 for 50ml

This rich but non-greasy product contains retinol and borage oil to aid cell renewal and leave the skin feeling soft. It also incorporates UV filters to prevent further damage from the sun.It melts into the skin, and is exquisitely scented.

■ LANCOME ABSOLUE NIGHT RECOVERY TREATMENT FOR NECK AND DECOLLETE

Best overnight treatment

£95 for 75ml

This nourishing cream is packed with wild yam, soya and sea algae to stimulate collagen and elastin production, resulting in stronger, more supple skin. It contains salicylic acid too to help lift away dead skin cells, leaving a clearer, more even skin.

■ LIERIC COHERENCE NECK FIRMING INTENSIVE LIFTING TREATMENT

Best product for younger skin

£40 for 50ml

This non-greasy gel-cream is formulated with active ingredients that encourage the skin's production of collagen, helping both to boost firmness and to prevent premature ageing. Skin is left softer and visibly lifted.

■ LIZ EARLE NATURALLY ACTIVE SKIN REPAIR

Best for all skin types

£10.50 for 50ml

Botanicals used in this treatment include echinacea, wheatgerm (rich in vitamin E) and borage oil. It can be used on the face and chest as well as the neck, and is available in versions for normal/combination and dry/sensitive skin.

EYE MAKE-UP REMOVERS

■ ACADEMIE DE BEAUTE HYPO-SENSITIVE EYE MAKE-UP REMOVER
Best for sensitive eyes
£15 for 250ml
This ultra-gentle gel is good for even the most sensitive eyes, and it even conditions the lashes as it cleanses.

■ AVEDA PURE GEL EYE MAKEUP REMOVER
Best natural remover for sensitive skin
£16 for 119ml
A gentle, non-greasy formula that uses coconut derivatives to dissolve eye make-up, lavender and echinacea to soothe delicate skin, and rosewater to refresh.

■ CHRISTIAN DIOR DUO-PHASE EYE MAKE-UP REMOVER
Best non-oily remover
£12.50 for 100ml
This fresh and non-oily lotion removes make-up gently yet effectively from the eyes. It needs to be shaken before use to mix the two levels.

■ CLARINS EYE MAKE-UP REMOVER
Best for conditioning lashes
£12 for 125ml
Plant extracts in this effective product include rosewater to calm and tone, cornflower to soothe, and soya protein to condition lashes.

■ CLINIQUE NATURALLY GENTLE EYE MAKEUP REMOVER
Best for contact lens wearers
£11 for 75ml
This is an extremely mild remover that contains a combination of natural ingredients resembling many of those found in tears, including a sugar-based natural emulsifier that works gently to dissolve and to remove eye make-up. As it leaves no greasy residue, it is suitable for contact lens wearers.

■ DERMALOGICA SOOTHING EYE MAKE-UP REMOVER
Best oil- and alcohol-free remover
£15.80 for 118ml
A gentle formula free of both oil and drying alcohol, this quickly removes all traces of eye make-up.

■ ESTEE LAUDER GENTLE EYE MAKE-UP REMOVER
Best gentle formula
£12 for 100ml
This lightweight, oil-free formula removes all forms of eye make-up without leaving any residue, making it suitable for contact lens wearers.

■ **LANCOME BI-FACIL**
Best for removing stubborn eye make-up
£15 for 125ml
Shake vigorously before use to disperse the oil particles suspended in the soothing blue fluid. This superb product removes even the most stubborn eye make-up. Especially good for contact lens wearers as it is non-irritating and gentle.

■ **L'OREAL PLENITUDE GENTLE EYE MAKE-UP REMOVER**
Best budget buy
£3.99 for 125ml
An excellent budget buy, this non-oily formula removes all traces of eye make-up without irritation and is enriched with pro-vitamin B5 to soothe and soften.

■ **PRESCRIPTIVES QUICK REMOVER FOR EYE MAKE-UP**
Best for soothing
£14 for 125ml
An oil-free and fragrance-free remover with cucumber extracts that is kind to sensitive eyes, while swiftly dissolving all traces of make-up.

■ **REN VITAMIN E EYE MAKE UP REMOVER**
Best pure remover
£13.50 for 150ml
A gentle but thorough lotion – over 97 per cent derived from plants and minerals – this contains soothing camomile and vitamin E to fight harmful free radicals.

■ **SISLEY GENTLE MAKE-UP REMOVER FOR EYES AND LIPS**
Best luxury remover
£22 for 125ml
Active botanical ingredients, including extracts of wild daisy, cornflower and gardenia, help to dissolve make-up in an instant while soothing lip and eye areas.

CLEANSERS

■ **AVON ANEW OXYGENATING CLEANSER**
Best for dull skins
£4 for 125ml
This fabulous product helps to breathe life into dull skin by increasing blood flow and oxygen delivery to the cells. It also contains milk protein, which moisturizes.

■ **CHRISTIAN DIOR REFRESHING CLEANSING WATER**
Best for normal skin
£14 for 200ml
This triple-action product gently cleanses and tones and removes eye make-up. It has a beautiful scent, makes cleansing ultra-quick and leaves skin feeling pure.

■ COSMETICS A LA CARTE TOTAL LIFT OFF

Best for make-up removal

£15 for 140g

The ingredients of this gentle, oil-free make-up remover include moisturizing aloe vera and calming rosewater to leave skin feeling fresh and ultra-cleansed. Make-up, pollution and mascara are removed in one easy sweep, resulting in clean, comfortable skin. Its gentle action also helps to exfoliate skin thereby preventing blocked pores and flakiness.

■ DECLEOR LAIT A DEMAQUILLER

Best botanical cleanser for all skin types

£14.50 for 250ml

This velvety-smooth cleansing milk is made up of plant extracts, including almond oil to soothe and lime flower water to hydrate, essential oils of lavender and petit grain to soften and smooth, and essential waters of orange, kiwi fruit and mallow. It gently removes make-up and eliminates impurities, while maintaining the skin's natural pH balance.

■ DERMALOGICA DERMAL CLAY CLEANSER

Best for calming, oily and acne-prone skin

£18.60 for 237ml

The natural clay in this cleanser removes excess oils, while extracts of cucumber and sage soothe irritation.

■ DR HAUSCHKA CLEANSING MILK

Best natural cleanser for sensitive skin

£16 for 150ml

Because of the oils of jojoba, almond and rice germ that it contains, this soothing, cleansing milk has a gentle, silky texture. (The plants and herbs used in Dr Hauschka's products are grown organically in rhythm with the phases of the moon and gathered just before sunrise when the life forces of the plants are strongest.) It seems to melt make-up, to leave skin thoroughly cleansed, soft and moisturized.

■ ELIZABETH ARDEN DEEP CLEANSING LOTION

Best for all skin types

£14 for 200ml

This cleansing lotion removes all impurities effectively without stripping the skin of moisture, so that all skin types are left clean and harmonized.

■ EVE LOM CLEANSING CREAM

Best deep cleanser

£39.50 for 100ml

Loved by models, actresses and beauty editors, this superlative cleanser is made from four aromatic oils and is removed with a specially woven muslin cloth. It is multifunctional, dissolving make-up, cleansing, toning and exfoliating the skin.

■ GUERLAIN ISSIMA FLOWER CLEANSING CREAM
Best for nourishing
£26 for 200ml

This is a rich one-step cleanser that removes even the most minute traces of make-up, even waterproof mascara, while at the same time nourishing and calming the skin. It has a lovely, soft floral scent, which is a result of the flower extracts that it contains – iris to purify, lily to soothe and rose to help totone the skin. Importantly, it also contains Calmitine-S, a valuable complex of protective active ingredients.

■ LANCOME EAU DE BIENFAIT CLARTE
Best cleanser and toner in one
£26 for 400ml

Packed with skin-nourishing vitamins, A and C for cell growth and radiance, and B5 and E for their soothing qualities, this cleanser will speed up your skincare routine, as it removes eye make-up, cleanses and tones in one go. It also contains pineapple enzymes and papaya which remove dead skin cells and give skin a fresh, healthy glow.

■ LAURA MERCIER ONE-STEP CLEANSER
Best for make-up removal and cleansing
£26 for 250g

This was devised by the make-up artist herself to remove even the most stubborn face and eye make-up, deep-cleanse and sweep away dead skin cells. It contains witch hazel, is moisturizing without drying, and readjusts the skin's PH balance.

■ MARIO BADESCU CLEANSING MILK WITH CARNATION & RICE OIL
Best for dry skin
£9.75 for 187g

An oil-based, milky cleanser that is recommended for dry or sensitive skin. The rich rice oil element prevents the skin from being stripped of moisture while it is being cleansed.

■ NASCENT FACIAL CLEANSER
Best for detoxifying
£16 for 125ml

All the ingredients in this effective organic cleanser are based on plants, so it's gentle enough for even sensitive skin types. It includes rose, rosemary, camomile and sandalwood (to help to detoxify) and ylang ylang (to regenerate the skin), and removes both make-up and environmental toxins.

■ NEUTROGENA DEEP CLEAN CREAM CLEANSER
Best budget buy
£4.25 for 200ml

This oil-free cleanser goes deep into pores, dissolving dirt, oil and make-up, and removing the dead skin cells that can dull the complexion.

■ REVLON ABSOLUTES CLARIFYING CLEANSING CREAM
Best for combination skin

£8.95 for 100ml

This balancing gel formula not only rids the skin of dirt and oil, but it also hydrates where it is needed at the same time, so it is highly effective for combination skin characterized by a greasy T-zone and dry cheeks.

■ SHISEIDO PURENESS DEEP CLEANSING FOAM
Best for blemish-prone or oily skin types

£15 for 100ml

This is a great product for deep-pore cleansing with oil control if you're prone to blemishes. The Pureness range contains syringa extract, which helps to reduce stress-hormone secretion, thus lessening the frequency of breakouts. If you wear make-up, use the Shiseido Pureness Cleansing Water first for best results.

FACE WASHES

■ CLARINS GENTLE FOAMING CLEANSER
Best for normal to oily skin

£13 for 125ml

A softly foaming cleanser, this is gentle yet effective enough to remove all impurities and make-up.

■ ESTEE LAUDER SPLASH AWAY FOAMING CLEANSER
Best for combination to oily skin

£14 for 150ml

A gentle but effective cream, this foaming cleanser penetrates the pores deeply and removes surface oil, dirt and make-up. It rinses off easily, leaving the skin feeling refreshed and soft, and maintains the skin's moisture balance so there is no dryness or tautness afterwards.

■ GARNIER SYNERGIE PURE GENTLE DEEP CLEAN FOAMING WASH
Best for young or spot-prone skin

£3.99 for 200ml

The rich, lathery foam washes away excess the oil and dirt that lead to spots, leaving skin superclean.

■ LIZ EARLE NATURALLY ACTIVE CLEANSE AND POLISH
Best for all skin types (including sensitive)

£10 for 100ml

Packed full of botanical ingredients including rosemary to stimulate circulation, hops to tone and soothe, and pure eucalyptus oil to purify, this highly effective cleanser is suitable for even sensitive skin. It is rinsed off with warm water and comes with its own muslin cloth to 'polish', or exfoliate, the skin.

■ L'OREAL PLENITUDE HYDRAFRESH FOAMING AND CLEANSING GEL

Best range for all skin types

£4.49 for 150ml

This light formula is soap-free, to prevent skin from drying out, and has added vitamins and minerals to leave the skin feeling healthy and fresh. It is offered in two formulations: for dry/sensitive and for normal/combination skin.

■ L'OREAL PURE ZONE DEEP EXFOLIATING GEL WASH

Best for oily or blemish-prone skin

£4.99 for 150ml

This clear, minty gel is wonderfully cooling and contains both the BHA salicylic acid to exfoliate gently and micro-beads to refine the complexion. Unlike many face washes designed specifically for spot-prone skin, it rinses off without irritating or drying out the skin.

FACIAL EXFOLIATORS

■ THE BODY SHOP MINERAL GENTLE EXFOLIATING MASK

Best for smoothing

£6 for 75ml

The fine grains in this rice-based scrub slough away dead skin cells to give an even complexion. This is definitely a good budget buy.

■ CLARINS ONE STEP EXFOLIATING CLEANSER

Best all-in-one exfoliator

£14.50 for 125ml

This rinse-off multipurpose product cleanses, tones, exfoliates and detoxifies the skin. Enriched with orange extract and moringa tree, it gently sloughs away dead skin cells with tiny micro beads, leaving skin feeling refreshed and toned.

TIPS

- If you suffer from dry skin and find using water makes the problem worse, choose cleansing creams that can be removed with tissues or cotton wool.
- Never cleanse the skin more than twice a day or you will risk stripping it of its natural moisture balance. This could eventually lead to such problems as flaky patches and excessive oil production.
- Wipe it out! Cleansing wipes that clean off eye make-up and tone skin are a handy product for the gym or to take on holiday.
- If you have particularly dry or sensitive skin, choose an exfoliator that contains synthetic granules rather than natural ones, such as rice. Synthetic granules are gentler and therefore less abrasive.

■ DERMALOGICA GENTLE CREAM EXFOLIANT
Best all-round exfoliator, improving skin's texture
£26.70 for 74ml
The hydroxyl acid complex removes dull surface cells, while conditioning botanical extracts and humectants soothe the skin and combat dryness. It is fragrance-free and thus suited to easily irritated faces.

■ ELEMIS GENTLE ROSE EXFOLIATOR
Best for sensitive or mature skin
£19.50 for 50ml
A light exfoliating gel containing rose oil and cucumber extract, this contains tiny jojoba beads for non-abrasive exfoliation. Gentle enough to use every day, it is ideal for smoothing and revitalizing sensitive and mature skin.

■ LABORATOIRE REMEDE SWEEP
Best deep-down exfoliator
£36 for 75ml
This is a paste of five white marble powders and clay that gives pores a clean sweep but which is gentle enough for even sensitive skin.

■ L'OCCITANE EXFOLIATING FACIAL MUD
Best for purifying skin
£14.95 for 100ml
Made with ground olive stones and olive oil, this richly textured, highly effective mud mask gently exfoliates and purifies, giving skin a glorious, healthy glow.

■ MURAD PURIFYING FACE SCRUB
Best for oily skin
£20.50 for 100ml
This gentle, yet effective facial scrub exfoliates and purifies skin at the same time. Kaolin works to absorb surface impurities while jojoba beads and cornmeal help to slough away dry, dull skin, to leave a smooth, polished skin.

■ ORIGINS NEVER A DULL MOMENT
Best for illuminating complexion
£20 for 125ml
This is a celebrity favourite that employs crushed papaya to dissolve old cells, while mango and ground apricot seeds gently polish the skin.

■ YVES SAINT LAURENT GOMMAGE BIOLOGIQUE INSTANT RADIANCE EXFOLIATOR
Best for softening
£28 for 75ml
A non-grainy, honey-textured gel, this product combines sugars that exfoliate the skin with oils that leave it soft and smooth. It is especially good for sensitive skin.

TONERS

■ AMANDA LACEY PERSIAN ROSEWATER
Best for sensitive skin
£32.50 for 250ml
Gentle and lightly hydrating, this exquisite toner rebalances skin naturally.
Rosewater is often recommended for sensitive skins as a gentler, natural
alternative to toners, which can sometimes be harsh.

■ BOBBI BROWN SOOTHING FACE TONIC
Best for refreshing all skin types
£15.50 for 200ml
This ultra-gentle toner contains a soothing blend of cucumber extract and
lavender. As it works so gently, it does not produce the tight feeling sometimes
prompted by cleansing but instead leaves the face refreshed and ready for
make-up or for bed.

■ CLARINS PURIFYING TONING LOTION
Best for balancing and calming
£13 for 200ml
Calming camomile and soothing cucumber combine with vitamins A, B and E
in this lotion to balance skin. A good tip is to keep a bottle in the fridge to use
when the weather is hot, as a wonderful means of cooling and freshening hot,
dry and flushed skin.

■ DERMALOGICA MULTI-ACTIVE TONER
Best for hydrating skin
£18.70 for 237ml
An ultra-light facial spritz that hydrates the skin while helping the absorption of
moisturizer. It contains soothing aloe vera blended with extracts of lavender and
arnica to condition and protect. It can be used to freshen up skin throughout
the day – even over make-up.

■ KIEHL'S ROSEWATER FACIAL FRESHENER-TONER
Best for normal to oily skin
£13.95 for 200ml
Complete with floating rose petals, this mildly astringent alcohol-free toner,
soothes and refreshes the skin delightfully.

■ MOLTON BROWN SKIN BALANCE TONING LOTION
Best for brightening skin
£ 17 for 200ml
This excellent, non-drying toner will exfoliate and brighten your complexion.
It contains pumpkin enzymes, a gentler alternative to AHAs, that help to remove
dead skin cells and leave skin feeling soft and revitalized.

BLEMISH TREATMENTS

◼ BENEFIT BOOBOO ZAP
Best quick-drying formula
£13.50 for 6ml
This clear, quick-drying blend of salicylic acid and camphor helps to take the redness from spots. The handy little bottle makes it easy to reapply as needed.

◼ BIORE BLEMISH BOMB
Best for reducing redness
£6.50 for 10 bombs
Place just one of these little capsules on a bad blemish and leave it overnight and by the morning it will have been magically reduced.

◼ CLINIQUE ANTI-BLEMISH SOLUTIONS CLEAR BLEMISH GEL
Best for speedy healing
£9.50 for 15ml
The salicylic acid in this clear gel helps to clear stubborn spots and speed healing.

◼ COSMETICS A LA CARTE ALL CLEAR
Best for treating blackheads
£15 for 40ml
This skin-tinted fluid tackles open pores, blackheads and spots. It is packed with antiseptic ingredients, such as tea tree, lavender and witch hazel, plus oil-blotting minerals to beat shine. Ideal as a foundation or an overnight intensive treatment.

◼ DERMALOGICA MEDICATED CLEARING GEL
Best medicated treatment gel
£24.90 for 59ml
Medicated salicylic acid contained in this gel acts as an exfoliating agent to help clear existing blemishes, while alginated zinc triplex gets deep into the pores and follicles to deep-cleanse, fight bacteria and regulate the production of sebum. Its botanical extracts and essential oils soothe and heal more troubled complexions.

◼ EVE LOM DYNASPOT
Best for calming angry spots
£16.50 for 9ml
The mixture of calamine, tea tree oil and mint in this natural yet powerful pink lotion calms spots overnight.

◼ LA PRAIRIE CELLULAR PURIFYING SYSTEME BLEMISH CONTROL
Best preventative spot cream
£40 for 15ml
An invisible, oil-free formula that not only targets spots and promotes healing, but also helps to prevent future flare-ups.

LIZ EARLE SPOT-ON
Best multipurpose treatment
£6.50 for 6ml
Packed with natural ingredients including tea tree oil, for its antiseptic properties, lavender to inhibit spots, and healing vitamin E, this product works quickly and comes in a handy airtight applicator. It is a potent, all-purpose remedy for blemishes, sores, cuts and bites.

MURAD MOISTURIZING ACNE TREATMENT GEL
Best for sore, spotty skin
£28.50 for 78ml
This lightweight, oil-free gel moisturizes skin at the same time that it is fighting spots, thereby helping to reduce redness and flakiness. Salicylic acid and retinol work together to manage breakouts, while tea tree oil soothes irritation and helps to prevent the development of further spots.

ORIGINS SPOT REMOVER
Best for diminishing irritation
£8.50 for 10ml
This clears up irritating spots in next to no time, thanks to its quick-acting natural ingredients, such as clove buds and oregano. Its invisible formula means that it can be worn during the day, under your normal make-up. For best results, apply as soon as you feel the blemish appearing.

OXY ON THE SPOT
Best for cleaning pores
£4.95 for 30ml
Containing benzoyl peroxide, this antibacterial product zaps spots rapidly by cleaning pores and encouraging skin to shed the dead cells that may block pores and result in spots.

PRESCRIPTIVES BLEMISH SPECIALIST
Best for soothing and controlling blemishes
£15 for 30ml
Ingredients in this blemish blitzer include oat extracts to soothe swelling and redness and Biodermine, a special soy protein extract that reduces surface oil. It works quickly and effectively, and contains a vital combination of acids to help prevent future breakouts.

PHYTOMER CORRIGEL
Best for reducing scarring
£15.50 for 30ml
This is a soothing gel that works to calm the skin and diminish inflammation while it is fighting spots as soon as they start to develop. It is designed to help reduce any redness and to prevent the scarring caused by blemishes.

■ **SHISEIDO PURENESS BLEMISH TARGETING GEL**
Best for minimizing spots
£15 for 15ml
This is an invisible, quickly absorbed gel that minimizes the appearance of blemishes while refreshing the skin.

■ **TISSERAND TEA TREE AND KANUKA BLEMISH STICK**
Best for fighting bacteria
£2.45 for 8ml
In a gel base that cleanses and soothes, pure essential oils of tea tree and kanuka work together to fight bacteria. A wand is supplied for precision application.

LIP TREATMENTS

■ **BLISSLABS BLISSBALM**
Best for moisturizing
£15 for 15g
This quickly absorbed, non-waxy but water-resistant balm contains antioxidant vitamin E in a moisture-binding beeswax base, to nourish even the driest lips.

■ **THE BODY SHOP BORN LIPPY**
Best for a touch of shine
£3 for 10ml
This balm comes in a range of different fruit flavours, so as well as adding moisture and shine, it tastes delicious!

■ **THE BODY SHOP LIPSCUFF**
Best for exfoliating
£5.50 for 4g
This is a useful product for sanding off any flaky skin on lips, before you apply balm or lipstick. Lips are left smooth and instantly more kissable.

■ **BURT'S BEES BEESWAX LIP BALM**
Best for nourishing
£3 for 8.5g
This bestselling beeswax balm is packed with soothing and nourishing natural ingredients to cure cracked lips.

■ **CAUDALIE GRAPESEED LIP CONDITIONER**
Best for sun protection and anti-ageing
£4 for 4g
Caudalie's products all contain grapeseed extract, a potent natural antioxidant. The creamy formula of this conditioner fills out any wrinkles, while UVA and UVB filters shield lips from harmful rays.

■ CLARINS LIP BEAUTY MULTI-TREATMENT
Best for hydrating
£10.50 for 2.6g
This is a long-lasting, rich treatment that hydrates the lips with olive oil, shea butter and moisturizing vitamin E.

■ EVE LOM KISS MIX
Best for revitalizing
£9.50 for 10ml
This rich, glossy formula moisturizes deeply and restores lips to peak kissing condition. Use on its own or over lipstick for added sheen.

■ KIEHL'S LIP BALM
Best for soothing and protecting
£6.50 for 15ml
A cult favourite with many models, this balm gives instant relief to dry, chapped lips. It contains soothing ingredients and moisturizing oils – a cold-weather must.

■ LANCASTER LIP CONDITIONING CREAM
Best for under lipstick
£20 for 15ml
While keeping lips soft and smooth, this cream provides a good base for lipstick. Ingredients such as glycerine, silicone wax and mineral oils protect and soothe.

■ MARTHA HILL PROTECTIVE LIP BALM
Best for softening
£5.50 for 15ml
This is a gentle balm that combines natural waxes, such as beeswax, with aloe vera, to soothe, and castor oil, to moisturize. Reapply at intervals throughout the day, because it contains a sunscreen which will provide additional protection.

■ NEAL'S YARD HERBAL LIP BALM
Best naturally based formula
£2.40 for 7.5g
This organic balm contains antioxidant vitamin E to nourish even the driest lips, and lavender essential oil for its soothing and antiseptic properties.

■ ORIGINS LIP REMEDY
Best intensive treatment
£7.50 for 5ml
Formulated specially as a treatment for cracked, chapped lips, this remedy includes menthol and camphor to soothe, French thyme and wintergreen oil to relieve dryness and roughness, and tea tree and olive oils to protect. It is absorbed rapidly and leaves no greasy after-feel, but it should be used only as long as the condition continues.

■ POUT INDULGE ME LIP BALM
Best for gloss and conditioning
£6 for 15ml
Shea butter has been blended with lavender in this smooth, glossy and sweet-smelling balm that is enriched with vitamins to keep lips in tip-top, kissable condition.

■ ULTIMA II EXTRAORDINAIRE VOLUMIZING LIP GLOSS (SPF 6)
Best for plumping
£13.50 for 5ml
Vitamin E, plus wheatgerm and sesame oils restore moisture and plump the lips, while light reflectors give maximum shine. Available in six shimmery shades, it also provides some sun protection.

■ VASELINE LIP THERAPY
Best for shine and all-over use
£1.15 for 20g
This classic, multipurpose petroleum balm is now available in a dinky tin. Vaseline is multifunctional, not only does it make lips soft and shiny but it can also be used for combating dry cuticles or adding a sheen to your eyelids and cheekbones – a handbag essential.

■ VICHY NUTRILOGIE LIPS
Best for dry, chapped lips
£3.50 for 40ml
If you suffer from dry, chapped lips during the winter, Vichy have your answer – used alone or under lipstick. Its active ingredients boost the production of lipids and collagen, which can be impaired when assaulted by wind, cold and UV rays.

BODY CLEANSERS

■ AVEDA ENERGIZING HAND AND BODY CLEANSER
Best botanical cleanser
£12 for 237ml
Aloe vera, grapefruit seed and witch hazel are just some of the natural ingredients in this effective botanical cleanser. With invigorating plant-derived aromas such as ylang ylang and peppermint, this will leave you feeling cleansed and refreshed.

■ CLINIQUE AROMATICS ELIXIR BODY WASH
Best for reviving
£17 for 200ml
If you're a fan of Clinique's Aromatics Elixir fragrance, you'll love this shimmery body wash. Used in the bath or shower, the gel leaves skin seductively scented with that distinctive blend of camomile, patchouli, ylang ylang, rose and jasmine.

■ DOVE CREAM BAR
Best budget soap

79p for 100g

We wouldn't generally recommend soap for skin but this is gentle enough for any skin type. Its unique composition, with 25 per cent moisturizing milk, leaves the skin soft, clean and comfortable. A sensitive version is also available.

■ E'SPA ESSENTIAL CLEANSING GEL
Best for sensitive skin

£14.95 for 250ml

An aromatic, soap-free cleansing gel, this is formulated with horse chestnut and soothing essential oils such as lavender and rose geranium. It leaves skin feeling soft and refreshed and is gentle enough to be used on the face.

■ FRESH HONEY FORMULA BATH FOAM
Best for hydrating

£17.50 for 300ml

Honey, a substance that has been renowned for centuries for its beauty-enhancing properties, is the key ingredient in this nourishing bath foam. It also features milk proteins and shea butter to hydrate and soften skin. Choose from three luscious scents – warm Honey Chestnut, fruity Honey Plum and fresh Honey Linden – or why not indulge in them all?

■ JO MALONE SHOWER GEL
Best for scent

£18 for 100ml

Unlike some shower gels, Jo Malone's range are surprisingly moisturizing, softly foaming and richly textured. As you would expect from this fragrance queen, they come in wonderful scents, including Nutmeg, Ginger and Grapefruit.

■ KIEHL'S LIQUID BATH AND SHOWER BODY CLEANSER
Best for all skin types

£13.50 for 200ml

This mild and pH-balanced liquid cleanser comes in a range of scents, including Mango, Peppermint and Vanilla. It rinses off easily, and leaves the skin silky smooth and fresh. Being pH balanced, it won't strip the skin of its natural oils.

■ KNEIPP JUNIPER HERBAL SHOWER AND BATH GEL
Best for tired bodies

£6.95 for 100ml

The blend of juniper with wintergreen oil in this gentle and yet effective natural gel helps to relieve tension, stimulate circulation and soothe tired muscles. You may also like to try Kneipp's other natural shower and bath gels, such as Lavender, Rosemary or Eucalyptus – which are just as effective for their stated purposes.

■ KORRES BASIL AND LEMON SHOWER GEL
Best for invigorating

£5 for 250ml

This foaming shower gel contains aloe vera and wheat proteins gently to cleanse and refresh the skin, and it wakes you up with a citrus zing.

■ LIZ EARLE ORANGE FLOWER BOTANICAL BODY WASH
Best for very sensitive skin

£9.50 for 200ml

An extremely gentle body wash, this is mild enough even for children. Orange flower water combines with essential oils of lavender, geranium and rosewood to leave the skin soft and smooth with a lovely, light fragrance.

■ L'OCCITANE AROMACHOLOGIE PURIFYING BATH
Best for purifying

£12.95 for 500ml

A marvellously relaxing bath oil with a rich foamy lather. It contains essential oils of lemon, cardamom and eucalyptus that help to rid the body of impurities and soothe the mind at the same time.

■ MARTHA HILL ROSE GERANIUM HARMONIZING BODY WASH
Best for relaxing

£5.80 for 200ml

Rose geranium oil, which is an excellent skin conditioner, and sweet orange and ylang ylang oils, which have a calming effect on the mind and body, are the crucial ingredients in this gentle, moisturizing body wash. It is also available as a bath oil for those who really want to unwind.

■ MOLTON BROWN BLISSFUL TEMPLETREE MOISTURE BATH AND SHOWER
Best for after sun

£12 for 300ml

This azure blue gel is beautifully scented with an infusion of fruit, marine and blossom extracts from Sri Lanka. It contains sea silk proteins from the Indian Ocean, to soothe skin after sun exposure, and mango oils and templetree (frangipani) milk to moisturize.

■ OLE HENRIKSEN CLARIFYING BODY WASH
Best herbal cleanser

£19.50 for 255ml

Developed by Hollywood skincare guru Ole Henriksen, this rich herbal body cleanser is simply brimming with fabulous ingredients. Amongst others, these include emollient comfrey, soothing camomile, and NAPCA, a natural humectant that seals in moisture. It leaves skin cleansed and silky, and is so gentle that it can even be used for babies' skin.

■ **ORIGINS A PERFECT WORLD CREAMY BODY CLEANSER WITH WHITE TEA**
Best for dry skin
£20 for 200ml
This luscious lathering cream cleanses the skin without washing away precious surface oils. Sweet orange oil, glycerine and shea butter help to guard against dryness, especially in problem areas like elbows and knees, while white tea works as an antioxidant.

■ **REN MONOI MOISTURIZING BODY RINSE**
Best for moisturizing
£15.95 for 150ml
This unique body-moisturizing formula is based on monoi oil, which has been used in Tahiti for centuries to keep skin supple. It's so effective that you won't need a body lotion, particularly with its delicate scent of tiare flowers.

■ **THE SANCTUARY BODY WASH**
Best for tense muscles
£3.99 for 250ml
This inexpensive yet effective cleanser uses a blend of essential oils and spices to help relieve tension, combined with sesame and jojoba oils to nourish skin.

BODY EXFOLIATORS

■ **AVEDA SMOOTHING BODY POLISH**
Best for smooth skin
£18 for 225g
The finely ground walnut shells in this creamy purifying foam gently polish your skin, while the extracts of kelp, aloe and lavender work to imbue it with a renewed smoothness.

■ **BIOTHERM POLISHING MUD EXFOLIATOR**
Best for revitalizing tired skin
New release, price TBC
This effective exfoliating mud contains extracts of algae and thermal plankton and is enriched with trace elements. Your body is left feeling totally revitalized and carrying a bracing aquatic scent.

■ **BLISS SPA LEMON PEEL BODY POLISHING SCRUB**
Best for invigorating
£20 for 240g
Use this invigorating citrus scrub before getting into the shower for a wonderful wake-up call for body and mind. Used regularly, you will find that even those dry patches on elbows and knees will respond.

■ CLINIQUE SOFT POLISH BODY EXFOLIATOR
Best for gentle exfoliation
£12.50 for 200ml
This peach-scented scrub contains the finest of granules; they resurface your skin without scratching it.

■ ELEMIS DEVIL'S MINT BODY SCRUB
Best for nourishing
£19.50 for 150ml
A fragrantly scented scrub, this is formulated with peppermint essential oil and a blend of sea plants such as Devil's Apron seaweed. It removes dead skin cells as it gently cleanses, nourishes and revitalizes skin.

■ E'SPA EXFOLIATING BODY POLISH
Best for deep cleansing
£25.50 for 200g
This rich, aloe-based gel contains extracts of spearmint, apricot kernel and phytoplankton. It is extremely effective and very thorough in its removal of impurities and dead skin cells.

■ ESTEE LAUDER CRYSTAL GLOW SUGAR RUB
Best for supersoft skin
£23 for 325g
Sugar cane has been blended with natural oils, such as those of sunflower and grapeseed, in a delectable rub that polishes away dead skin and flakiness and rehydrates dry skin.

■ FRESH BROWN SUGAR BODY POLISH
Best for stimulating circulation
£47 for 435g
A delicious blend of pure sugar and fine oils, this exfoliator removes toxins and improves circulation to leave skin renewed, sweet-smelling and glowing.

■ GUERLAIN ISSIMA BLUE EXFOLIATING SCRUB
Best for dry skin
£22.50 for 150ml
This rich, delicious-smelling cream contains exfoliating grains and seashell powder to help smooth rough spots and revitalize the skin, and hydrating agents which will prevent skin from drying out.

■ HELENA RUBINSTEIN SWEET SUGAR BODY SCRUB
Best for sensitive skin
£22 for 200ml
This exfoliator contains very refined sugar granules so it is gentle and suitable even for sensitive skin. It is sweetly scented and doesn't leave an oily residue.

■ KANEBO FOAMING BODY EXFOLIATOR
Best for moisturizing
£24.95 for 250ml
Spherical silica polishing grains are combined with high-potency moisturizers and green tea extract to leave skin silky smooth.

■ L'OCCITANE VERBENA EXFOLIATING SALTS
Best for refreshing
£19.95 for 500g
Mediterranean sea salts are blended with sweet almond, apricot and grapeseed oils in this gentle exfoliator that refreshes skin leaving it delicately perfumed.

■ L'OREAL PLENITUDE EXFOTONIC
Best for rough patches
£8.99 for 200ml
This uplifting, citrus-scented scrub with AHAs and crystals tackles even roughest of patches on the elbows, knees and ankles. Not suitable for sensitive skin.

■ NEAL'S YARD SEAWEED SALT SCRUB
Best natural product
£13.25 for 150g
This invigorating scrub combines clays and mineral-rich seaweeds to improve skin tone with Dead Sea salts to exfoliate and help remove toxins. It also contains patchouli, lemon and grapefruit essential oils to stimulate skin, and glycerine and avocado oils to leave it smooth and soft.

■ ORIGINS SALT RUB SMOOTHING BODY SCRUB
Best for scent
£25 for 600g
A celebrity favourite, this scrub contains mineral-rich Dead Sea salts buffered in macadamia, soya bean and sweet almond oils to silken skin. And it's scented with reviving spearmint and rosemary.

■ PHILOSOPHY AMAZING GRACE OLIVE OIL BODY SCRUB
Best for long-term protection
£14.50 for 473.1g
Not only does this give the benefit of deep cleansing with Dead Sea salts, but your skin is also protected and moisturized by the emollient properties of olive oil.

■ YVES SAINT LAURENT GOMMAGE ACTION BIOLOGIQUE
Best for renewing
£26 for 100ml
The papaya, microscopic pearls and sugars in this exfoliator work effectively to remove dead skin cells. The extracts of lemon and Asian citrus fruits packed with vitamin C, fruit acids and pectins help to promote renewal and hydration.

BODY MOISTURIZERS

■ AVEDA ROSEMARY MINT BODY LOTION
Best for invigorating benefits
£18 for 200ml
Invigorating and energizing, this lightweight, cooling lotion is made of organic plant-derived ingredients, such as organic aloe vera to soothe, corn starch, antioxidizing vitamins A and E, and rosemary for stimulating freshness.

■ THE BODY SHOP BODY BUTTER
Best for very dry skin
£10 for 200ml
These non-greasy body butters are delectable for dehydrated skin, especially during the winter. They are available in ten mouthwatering varieties, including Blueberry, Mango, Honey, Olive and Coconut.

■ BLISS SPA LEMON AND SAGE BODY BUTTER
Best for feeling pampered
£20 for 250ml
Deeply moisturizing, this deliciously scented product leaves dry skin baby soft and freshly scented. Massage this in and you'll feel as if you've been pampered for hours.

■ CLARINS BODY TREATMENT OIL 'RELAX'
Best for tired bodies
£27.50 for 100ml
Comprising 100 per cent pure plant extracts and aromatic oils, this is the ideal stress-busting, moisturizing treatment after exercise or if you're feeling run-down.

■ CLINIQUE SOOTHING WRAP BODY OIL
Best for relaxing
£14 for 200ml
Sesame and coconut palm oils are combined with essential oils of lavender, coriander and orange in this nourishing and relaxing body moisturizer. It can also be used as a massage oil or relaxing bath oil.

■ DECLEOR SYSTEME CORPS MOISTURIZING BODY MILK
Best for hydrating
£22 for 250ml
This light-textured lotion leaves skin hydrated and velvety smooth.

■ ESTEE LAUDER RESILIENCE LIFT BODY LOTION
Best for mature skin
£28 for 200ml
Replenishing, smoothing and hydrating, this moisturizer contains Estee Lauder's 'body lift complex' to help boost natural collagen production.

■ GATINEAU BODY LOTION WITH AHA
Best for normal to dry skin
£22 for 400ml
Vegetable proteins help rehydrate, while malic acid (an AHA derived from apples) wrapped in soya lipids ensures the skin is toned and refined without any irritation.

■ GUERLAIN ISSIMA BODY SUPER AQUA SERUM
Best for luminous skin
£40 for 150ml
Rich but non-greasy, this exquisite lotion contains 'blue gold' (Guerlain's exclusive blend of pure gold and oil extracted from marine algae), alongside other anti-ageing ingredients such as shea butter, to leave skin luminous and ultra-soft.

■ JO MALONE LIME, BASIL AND MANDARIN BODY LOTION
Best for all skin types
£20 for 100ml
The perfect summer moisturizer, this is light yet effective and smells deliciously fresh. Her fragrances can be combined and layered to create scents individual to you.

■ KIEHL'S CREME DE CORPS
Best for nourishing
£15 for 100ml
A cult favourite with models, this luxurious custard-like body lotion is enriched with betacarotene to nourish and moisturize even the driest skin.

■ KORRES GUAVA BODY BUTTER
Best for rough skin
£9 for 150ml
With natural ingredients, including guava, shea butter, quince extract and sunflower, almond and avocado oils, this ultra-rich body butter provides intense moisturizing. Especially good for rough areas like the elbows, knees and ankles.

■ LA PRAIRIE CELLULAR BUFFING OIL
Best luxury moisturizer
£59 for 200ml
This extra-light oil formulation is rich in marine nutrients and natural oils, plus essential oils of bergamot to stimulate and nutmeg to soothe. Massage this in during and after a bath or shower, to leave skin looking and feeling younger.

■ LANCOME AROMATONIC ENERGIZING BODY LOTION
Best for energizing
£20.50 for 200ml
Infused with refreshing essential oils such as lime, cardamom and ginger, this invigorating lotion is also packed with nourishing vegetable oils and vitamin E to soothe skin. Try the shower gel and body spritz, too, for the full experience!

LIZ EARLE ENERGIZING HIP AND THIGH GEL
Best for sluggish or puffy skin
£19.50 for 200ml
Containing ten pure essential oils plus herbal extracts in a base of organic damask rosewater, this gel is absorbed quickly into the skin and helps to eliminate toxins. It's seriously good for cellulite.

L'OCCITANE HONEY BODY BALM
Best for sensitive skin
£22.50 for 250ml
A luscious moisturizer containing natural honey and royal jelly to calm and hydrate the skin. This is a soothing treat for sensitive skin.

NEUTROGENA BODY OIL
Best for all-over moisture
£6.99 for 250ml
This natural oil, with a sesame seed oil base, soaks so well into the skin that it won't leave as much as a trace on your clothes.

NIVEA BODY SKIN FIRMING LOTION Q10
Best for firming
£5.49 for 200ml
The antioxidant co-enzyme Q10 along with liposomes carrying natural safflower oil help to improve the skin's firmness and leave it soft and smooth to the touch. This lotion is tremendous value for money.

ORIGINS GLOOM AWAY GRAPEFRUIT BODY SOUFFLE
Best for normal to oily skin
£20 for 200ml
This light and fluffy cream leaves skin feeling silky and smelling delicious. As the name predicts, the uplifting citrus scent will cheer you up on dark days.

PRADA HYDRATING BODY CREAM
Best fragrance-free product
£45 for 100ml
This fragrance-free cream sinks in quickly and gives you skin that is fit to set flashbulbs popping at a Prada fashion show. What is more, not only is this a great cream but the packaging looks beautiful in your bathroom, too.

SPACE NK BODY BALM 'ENRAPTURE'
Best for scent
£17 for 200ml
An intensive moisturizing balm full of skin nourishers such as shea butter and evening primrose and almond oils, this lives up to its name. The sensuous scent of tuberose will send you into raptures.

▪ Z BIGATTI CASHMERE BODY LOTION
Best for anti-ageing benefits

£110 for 113g

This luscious body lotion was formulated by world renowned US dermatologist Jennifer Bigelow. Containing vitamin complex, enzymes, botanical extracts, AHAs, and with anti-ageing properties, it exfoliates, refines and firms skin all over.

HAND TREATMENTS

▪ ATRIXO REGENERATING TREATMENT
Best budget buy

£3.79 for 75ml

A rich formula that is absorbed surprisingly quickly, this treatment uses liposome technology to deliver active ingredients that help to soothe rough, dry skin and reduce the prominence of age spots. An excellent budget buy, it comes in an easy-to-use dispenser and has a pleasant smell.

▪ BLISSLABS GLAMOUR GLOVES
Best for overnight hand treatment

£36 for a pair

The special polymer-gel lining in these unique gloves treats dry hands with moisturizing vitamin E and grapeseed, jojoba and olive oils. For a complete spa-style treatment, work the Glamour Glove Gel into the hands first, before putting on the gloves and drifting off to sleep.

▪ CHRISTIAN DIOR PROTECTIVE NOURISHING CREAM FOR HANDS (SPF 8)
Best for moisturizing

£11 for 75ml

A ceramide-rich moisturizing complex that leaves hands velvety soft while also offering some sun protection.

▪ CIRCAROMA ROSE HAND THERAPY CREAM
Best for sensitive skin

£15 for 120g

This is an entirely natural cream made with organic rosewater, rose attar and geranium, plus richly moisturizing shea butter. It smells heavenly.

▪ CLARINS HAND AND NAIL TREATMENT CREAM
Best for everyday use

£14 for 100ml

This multitasker softens hands with shea butter, strengthens nails with myrrh extract and minimizes brown spots on the backs of hands caused by sun damage with Japanese mulberry extract.

■ CRABTREE & EVELYN'S GARDENER'S HAND RECOVERY
Best for dry and rough hands
£12.50 for 100ml

If you're an avid gardener or regularly suffer from dry hands, this great all-in-one exfoliator and moisturizer is meant for you. Moisturizing ingredients include shea butter to keep skin soft and supple, plus botanical extracts of clover, marigold and yarrow to soothe.

■ DERMALOGICA MULTIVITAMIN HAND AND NAIL TREATMENT (SPF 15)
Best for hands and nails
£15.30 for 74ml

An intense yet non-greasy cream, this treatment boasts pro-vitamin B5 and algae extracts to repair and protect dry hands, and sweet almond oil to strengthen brittle nails against splitting and peeling. It also contains liquorice extract, vitamin C and good sun protection to prevent skin damage and signs of ageing.

■ DR HAUSCHKA HAND CREAM
Best natural cream for dry or sensitive skin
£8 for 50ml

This naturally-based product contains pure plant oils (almond, peanut, jojoba and wheatgerm) plus glycerine and extracts of marshmallow and carrot – to help heal cracks and dryness in worn-out hands. All ingredients in Dr Hauschka products are organic and biodynamically grown, so they are suitable for sensitive skin.

■ FRESH SOY HAND CREAM
Best for revitalizing and moisturizing
£19.50 for 75ml

A silky white cream that is instantly absorbed, a blend of beneficial soy proteins with ginseng, comfrey, shea butter, mango butter, glycerine and beeswax. It is a gentle cream that soothes and leaves hands feeling cool and refreshed.

■ GATINEAU VITAMIN A SURACTIF HAND CREAM
Best for supersoft hands
£11.50 for 100ml

A rich formula that sinks easily into the skin, this hand cream contains anti-ageing ingredients including a sunscreen and vitamins A and E to help fight free radicals, plus a complex of sugar derivatives to leave skin supple and soft. If skin is very dry, apply thickly and leave on the hands as a mask for 15-20 minutes.

■ JURLIQUE LAVENDER HAND CREAM
Best natural cream
£14.45 for 40ml

This rich yet non-greasy cream employs honey, soya lecithin, macadamia and lavender to soften even the driest hands and give them a heavenly aroma.

■ **KANEBO SENSAI INTENSIVE HAND TREATMENT**

Best for healing properties

£54.95 for 100ml

An oriental infusion is the magic ingredient that encourages the rehydration
and healing of neglected and overworked hands.

■ **LA PRAIRIE CELLULAR HAND CREAM**

Best for anti-ageing

£48 for 100ml

This luxurious cream provides intensive moisturization and contains marine-
derived AHAs that slough away flaky skin, leaving hands noticeably smoother.

■ **LANCASTER SURACTIF RETINOL 'DEEP LIFT' AGE PROTECTION
HAND CREAM (SPF 12)**

Best for sun protection

£25 for 100ml

Contains retinol, vitamin E and glycerine to soften, and a protective UV sun filter.

■ **LIZ EARLE HAND REPAIR**

Best for scent

£7.50 for 50ml

Packed with antioxidants, plus vitamin B to soften, this sinks in fast to leave skin
seriously soft and scented with soothing lavender, bergamot and camomile.

■ **L'OCCITANE HAND CREAM**

Best for retaining moisture

£12.95 for 150ml

Rich but non-greasy and easily absorbed, this bestselling product contains 20 per
cent shea butter as well as nourishing almond, honey, linseed and coconut oils.

■ **ROC RETINOL ACTIF PUR HAND CREM**

Best for minimizing age spots

£9.95 for 50ml

This non-greasy cream contains a sunscreen and retinol to bleach brown spots
and fade wrinkles, and vitamins B5 and E and glycerine to moisturize.

NAIL TREATMENTS

■ **CREATIVE NAIL DESIGN SOLAR OIL**

Best for dry cuticles

£8.25 for 14.79ml

This wonder-product contains a blend of vitamin E, rice bran and almond oil – to
soften the cuticles while strengthening nails. Simply massage this supernourishing
oil into the nail each night before going to bed. It smells gorgeously nutty, too.

■ DECLEOR AROMESSENCE ONGLES NAIL TREATMENT OIL
Best for luxury treatment
£30.50 for 15ml
Essential oils of myrrh, lemon and parsley are blended in a base of castor, hazelnut and avocado oils. Massage into the base of nails daily.

■ DR HAUSCHKA NEEM NAIL OIL
Best natural treatment for brittle nails
£18 for 30ml
Use a couple of drops of this wonderful natural oil every day to regenerate weak nails. Massaging it in well, combined with regular use, will promote strong, healthy nail growth and keep cuticles in great condition.

■ JESSICA PHENOMEN OIL
Best multipurpose treatment
£11.40 for 148ml
This blend of oils contains jojoba for healing dry, split and cracked cuticles, together with almond and rice oils to condition nails. Being a multipurpose product it is extremely flexible and can also be used to hydrate other problem areas such as elbows, feet and knees.

■ LIZ EARLE SUPERBALM
Best intensive treatment
£12.30 for 30g
Made of wholly natural ingredients, this miracle balm transforms even the driest hands, nails and cuticles. It sinks in astonishingly quickly.

■ NAILTIQUES NO 2
Best for weak nails
£15.95 for 14.8ml
Use this daily strengthener to cure soft, flaky nails. It contains protein to help bond split or peeling nails, helping them to grow long, strong and healthy.

■ OPI NAIL ENVY
Best for brittle nails
£14.95 for 15ml
The hydrolysed wheat protein, vitamin E and calcium in this product work to improve weak, brittle nails. It makes nails stronger without losing flexibility. Use the treatment as a base or top coat for maintenance.

■ PHILOSOPHY SAVE THE NAILS
Best for rough cuticles
£11 for 14.2g
Apply this vitamin-rich salve every day to keep cuticles in check. It contains calcium and folic acid to feed nails and encourage strong, healthy growth.

■ REVIVANAIL
Best for weak nails
£9.95 for 30ml
Containing formaldehyde to help promote stronger, longer and healthier nails, it works best if you apply one coat each day for a week, and then remove.

■ SALLY HANSEN AHA CUTICLE REMOVER AND CONDITIONER
Best for split or peeling nails
£3.95 for 13.3ml
The fruit acids in this product gently exfoliate dry, rough cuticles and help to condition split or peeling nails.

■ SALLY HANSEN NON-ACETONE NAIL POLISH REMOVER
Best gentle polish remover
£1.99 for 2.37ml
This remover is acetone-free so it won't strip nails of their natural oils. It also contains vitamin E and camomile to help care for and protect the nails.

■ SHU UEMURA NAIL CARE HYDRATING BASE COAT
Best for dry nails
£10 for 10ml
Pro-vitamin B5 and moisturizing ceramides worl together to keep cuticles moist and give nails a sleek, all-over gloss.

■ SPACE NK NAIL POLISH REMOVER
Best enriching polish remover
£6.50 for 100ml
Containing castor seed oil, sweet almond oil and vitamin E, this acetone-free formula efficiently removes polish without stripping nails of their vital oils.

FOOT AND LEG TREATMENTS

■ AVEDA FOOT RELIEF
Best for tired feet
£15 for 125ml
Botanical ingredients such as lavender, rosemary oil and jojoba soothe and deodorize while natural fruit acids (salicylic and lactic) soften even the toughest skin. An invigorating minty smell wafts up delightfully from the ground.

■ BENEFIT BATHINA SANDAL SCANDAL MOISTURIZER
Best for dry feet
£27.50 for 130ml
Packaged in a gorgeously kitsch 1950s-style pot, this is formulated with 10 per cent AHAs to remove any rough patches and make feet silky smooth.

■ BLISSLABS SOFTENING SOCKS
Best overnight treatment for feet
£36 for a pair
For best results rub Blisslabs Softening Sock Salve into your feet first before putting on these special socks and leaving them on overnight. You will wake up in the morning with sublimely soft soles.

■ THE BODY SHOP PEPPERMINT COOLING FOOT LOTION
Best for soothing
£5.50 for 250 ml
A budget beauty classic that softens hard heels and contains peppermint oil and menthol to soothe and revive tired feet.

■ BURT'S BEES FOOT CREAM
Best for healing
£8.95 for 113g
An ultra-rich, luxurious foot cream that contains beeswax, olive oil, coconut oil and vitamin E. This foot cream is guaranteed to soothe and soften even the driest and most overworked feet, smoothing hard skin, healing cracks and soothing sores along the way.

■ CAKE BEAUTY CAKE WALK TRIPLE MINT FOOT CREME
Best for after exercise
£11.50 for 120ml
An indulgent cream, this is made of nourishing avocado oil, mango butter and spearmint. Rough skin and tired feet soon become a thing of the past.

■ CLARINS ENERGIZING LEG EMULSION
Best for tired legs
£17.50 for 125ml
This is an instant pick-me-up for overworked legs and feet. For mothers-to-be or those who stand on their feet all day, this soothing treatment will enliven the legs.

■ CRABTREE & EVELYN FOOT BRUSH WITH PUMICE
Best tool for rough feet
£5.50
Natural pumice stone is ideal for sloughing away rough patches from the heels and the soles of the feet.

■ DECLEOR COMFORT FOOT CREAM
Best for refreshing feet
£14.75 for 50ml
Rich in plant extracts to help to purify and rebalance, thereby preventing excessive foot perspiration. This soothing cream is oil-free and easily absorbed so feet are not left feeling slippery.

■ ELIZABETH ARDEN GREEN TEA GRITTY FOOT POLISH
Best for exfoliating
£10 for 200ml
Refreshingly scented with green tea, this scrub contains pumice to buff away dead skin. Moisturize afterwards for silky feet.

■ ESTEE LAUDER SMOOTHING FEAT MANICURE/PEDICURE TREATMENT
Best for dry feet and hands
£15 for 250ml
An intensely hydrating treatment with rich emollients, this will treat rough feet or dry hands literally in minutes.

■ KNEIPP ARNICA LEG SPRAY
Best for aching legs
£4.99 for 100ml
A cooling leg tonic that helps to relieve and relax tired, swollen or aching legs. Arnica is a natural anti-inflammatory and has a great effect on sprains and bruises, making this an excellent product to use after sport.

■ MARTHA HILL ENERGIZING LEG GEL
Best for sore muscles and swelling
£8.90 for 100ml
This revitalizing treatment gel contains seaweed complex and witch hazel, plus toning and relaxing oils of lime and peppermint. It massages in easily and is readily absorbed, helping to relieve sore muscles and reduce swellings.

■ NAILTIQUES AVOCADO FOOT CREAM
Best for nourishing
£13.95 for 114g
This deep-penetrating, non greasy moisturizer is specially formulated with nourishing avocado to condition rough, dry feet.

■ NEAL'S YARD COMFREY AND MALLOW FOOT BALM
Best natural treatment
£6.95 for 40g
Skin-softening almond and wheatgerm oils are blended with soothing extracts of marshmallow, marigold and comfrey to make this revitalizing treat for tired feet.

■ OLE HENRIKSEN FOOT FETISH ANTI-FATIGUE FOOT AND LEG LOTION
Best for tired feet and legs
£4.25 for 355ml
An energizing mix of peppermint, geranium and lavender oils, plus soothing seaweed extract, is the secret of this lovely lotion. Massage it into feet and legs in long, firm strokes night and morning.

■ ORIGINS SOLE SEARCHER

Best for rough feet

£12.50 for 150ml

Peppermint, pumice (lava rock), sandalwood, lemon and nutmeg work together in this foot scrub to alleviate dryness and to transform rough soles into velvet. Apply to damp soles and heels, then massage in a circular motion to smooth and soften tough skin layers.

■ PHILOSOPHY SOUL OWNER

Best for softening

£11 for 93.6g

This ultra-rich pampering foot cream contains glycolic and salicylic acids to slough away dead skin, leaving rough feet soft. Great for people who do a lot of walking and build up hard skin on their feet.

BUST CREAMS

■ BODY ULTIMATE BUST FIRMING GEL

Best for smoothing skin

£17.95 for 250ml

This is a highly effective product if you long for your bust to be perkier and silky smooth. When you use the rich blend of cedarwood, lemongrass and petitgrain the lifting effect is instant, the skin tone enhanced and the breast area plumped.

■ CLARINS BUST BEAUTY LOTION

Best for mothers-to-be

£27.50 for 50ml

The best product for preventing stretch marks during pregnancy. A combination of toning ginseng and nourishing olive extracts keep skin firm, supple and mark-free. Use morning and night for best results.

■ LIERAC BUST LIFT FIRMING SPRAY

Best for skin brightening

£21 for 100ml

This intensive treatment boosts skin tone and combats signs of dryness. The handy spray contains organic silicon and wheatgerm to maintain moisture levels, while gentle AHAs remove dead skin cells, revealing fresher, younger-looking skin.

■ MATIS BUST GEL TONIC

Best for mature skins

£16.60 for 125ml

Particularly good for older skin, this cream tightens and tones the breast area. A mixture of wheat proteins and wakame – a form of seaweed rich in amino acids – keeps skin moisturized, while sweet almond oil nourishes and protects.

■ PHYTOMER INTENSIVE BUST GEL
Best for preventing sagging
£23 for 50 ml

This non-greasy gel is easily absorbed and, as it rehydrates, it improves the elasticity of skin around the bust and décolletage, helping to minimize drooping..

■ SISLEY BOTANICAL INTENSIVE BUST COMPOUND
Best intensive treatment
£82 for 50ml

This is great to use as an uplifting treatment post-pregnancy, to help strengthen the skin's natural support system. It is rich in natural toning ingredients, such as horsetail, ivy, and yarrow, which work quickly on the contours of your bust.

CELLULITE TREATMENTS

■ BLISSLABS HIGH THIGHS SUPPORT SERUM
Best for lifting
£29 for 150ml

This light gel is absorbed instantly. Packed with marine minerals and antioxidants it helps boost elasticity, breaks down fatty deposits and prevents stretch marks. Used regularly, the skin feels firmer and the appearance of cellulite is reduced.

■ CHRISTIAN DIOR BIKINI TONICITE BODY CONTOURING AND TONING CONCENTRATE
Best for smoothing
£28 for 200ml

An ultra-fine, spray-on emulsion, this penetrates quickly to tackle cellulite, water retention and lack of firmness. Dior claims that your silhouette should be noticeably toned and streamlined within a month.

■ DECLEOR LIFT CELLUMIUM ANTI-CELLULITE SLIMMING GEL
Best for refining
£25.75 for 150ml

This slimming gel helps to break down fat pockets, disperse excess water and diminish dimpling, and refine the figure. Its ingredients include algae, butcher's broom extract and one per cent AHAs to smooth and hydrate the skin's surface.

■ ELEMIS CELLUTOX ACTIVE BODY CONCENTRATE
Best for detoxifying
£26.50 for 100ml

Superstars in this 100 per cent botanical firming product include sea fennel, juniper and lemon, in a base of moisturizing almond and sunflower oils. Quick-penetrating and surface-smoothing, it aims to reduce the appearance of cellulite and helps to rid the body of toxins. DO NOT use when pregnant or breast-feeding.

■ GARNIER BODY TONIC CONTOUR FIRMING GEL
Best value-for-money treatment
£8.99 for 150ml
This is an oil-in-water emulsion with a blend of fruit essences – selected for their stimulating properties – and caffeine. Non-greasy, it is instantly absorbed and aims to decrease cellulite by refining the body's contours.

■ GATINEAU REACTIV'R SLENDERIZING EMULSION GEL
Best for boosting circulation
£25 for 200ml
This blue-green gel contains alcohol, menthol and a cooling agent to gently boost the circulation, an algae-derived complex to strengthen the collagen and elastin fibres in the skin and caffeine to stimulate. Its aim is to firm and tone dimply skin, greatly reducing the appearance of cellulite.

■ L'OREAL PLENITUDE BODY EXPERTISE PERFECT SLIM
Best for reducing the orange-peel effect
£10.99 for 200ml
A firming and contouring body gel that is formulated with caffeine, known for its stimulating properties, gingko, to help tone and boost the skin's tissues and Par-Elastyl, an active firming agent. L'Oreal claims that it improves the appearance of 'orange-peel' skin as well as smoothing and toning the body.

■ PHYTOMER SEATONIC BODY FIRMING CREAM
Best for firming and toning
£28.50 for 250ml
Succharide, a brown algae complex, is one of the main ingredients used in this non-greasy firming body cream. When it is applied directly after bathing, it helps to prevent the skin from sagging by protecting and restructuring the collagen and elastin fibres.

■ SISLEY PHYTO SCULPTURAL ANTI-CELLULITE
Best for severe cellulite
£57 for 150ml
This easily absorbed gel-emulsion is packed with active plant-based extracts, including extract of bitter orange and soy. It also contains caffeine, horse chestnut and essential oils of rosemary and lavender. Its aim is to slim, drain and firm. Sisley claims that when it was tested by 100 women, 90-98 per cent of them noticed a visible result.

■ YVES SAINT LAURENT LIGNE PURE
Best for improving skin tone
£32.50 for 200ml
With active ingredients including bitter orange, caffeine and marine plankton, this should improve skin tone after just eight days of twice-daily massage.

FAKE TANS

■ CHRISTIAN DIOR GOLDEN SELF TANNER INSTANT GLOW FOR THE FACE
Best for instant glow
£16 for 50ml
Gentle self-tanner that gives an immediate glow to the face. Will not block pores.

■ CLARINS RADIANCE PLUS SELF TANNING CREAM GEL
Best non-sticky formula
£21.50 for 50ml
Vitamins A and E, pro-vitamin B5 and minerals enrich the skin while two self-tanning ingredients work in tandem to bring out an even, impressive bronze colour.

■ CLARINS SELF TANNING INSTANT SPRAY
Best spray
£14 for 150ml
This invisible mist develops into a really natural-looking tan in a couple of hours.

■ CLINIQUE SELF-SUN QUICK BRONZE
Best oil-free formula
£12 for 125ml
An oil-free self-tanner that bronzes the skin immediately with a slight shimmer, it later develops into a long-lasting tan.

■ DECLEOR EXPRESS SELF-TAN (SPF 6)
Best DHA-free fake tan
£17.50 for 150ml
A light, milky-textured, instant-drying spray that uses organic mahakanni to develop a natural-looking, long-lasting tan in one hour. Decléor self-tanners are free of DHAs, which can irritate sensitive skin and tend to have a drying effect.

■ ELEMIS TOTAL GLOW SELF TANNING CREAM
Best for face and body
£19 for 125ml
Easily absorbed, this self-tanning treatment gives a natural-looking golden tan within two to three hours. Contains Instabronze, which helps to stimulate melanin production; antioxidant macadamia nut oil; vitamin E to help protect skin from harmful free radicals; and milk protein to nourish.

■ ESTEE LAUDER GO BRONZE TINTED SELF-TANNER
Best for a deep tan
£16.50 for 150ml
Tinted for foolproof application, this body bronzer gives an instant glow that lasts for days. It is also available in a formulation for the face.

■ ESTEE LAUDER SELF ACTION SUPER TAN SPRAY
Best clear formula
£15 for 125ml
Oil-free self-tanning mist comes in a handy spray that twists in any direction for easy application. It gives a natural-looking bronze tan in under two hours that lasts a day.

■ GARNIER AMBRE SOLAIRE NO STREAKS BRONZER SELF-TANNING SPRAY
Best value for money
£8.99 for 125ml
Creates a golden, even tan and gives a little sun protection on the beach as well. The formula will develop smoothly without streaking or a muddy effect.

■ KANEBO HONEY RADIANT SELF TANNING GEL
Best for hydrating and tanning
£24.95 for 200ml
Among the main ingredients in this product are purified honey to moisturize, sage extract to help to reduce the risk of skin damage, and silk extract to promote smoothness. It gives a glossy, bronze tan and has a clean, pleasant scent.

■ LANCASTER TINTED INSTANT SELF TAN BRONZER (SPF 4)
Best for moisturizing
£14.50 for 50ml
This light tinted gel, which takes only an hour to develop, gives a soft glow to the skin. It contains an SPF 4 as well as a moisturizing complex to hydrate the skin.

■ LANCOME FLASH BRONZER INSTANT SELF TANNING BODY SPRITZ
Best body spray
£17 for 150ml
Easy-to-use, this spray that dries almost instantly and has a non-oily feel, so you can dress without risk quite soon after applying it. The tan it produces in less than an hour is an even, convincing colour.

TIPS

- Always exfoliate skin before applying a self-tan product, paying particular attention to the knees, elbows and ankles – these drier areas can absorb too much product and make the tan look patchy.
- Don't moisturize before application unless the instructions specifically direct you to do so. It can dilute the product and lead to an uneven finish.
- Once your fake tan has been applied, moisturize on a daily basis after showering and bathing to make it last longer.
- Use a self-tan product specifically designed for the face – body products tend to contain more oil, which can block pores on the face.

■ LANCOME FLASH BRONZER TINTED SELF TANNING FACE CREAM-GEL (SPF 15)
Best for the face
£17 for 50ml

Light-reflecting pearls enhance the complexion immediately and a deep natural tan develops within an hour. Enriched with vitamin E and honey, this cream-gel leaves the face soft, will not clog pores and has a valuable SPF 15.

■ L'OREAL PLENITUDE SUBLIME BRONZE EXPRESS BODY
Best for a smooth, even tan
£9.99 for 150ml

This self-tanning spray creates a natural-looking, non-orange tan that lasts for a long time. The gentle AHA formula smooths the skin for an even tan, and moisturizes for up to 12 hours.

■ NIVEA TOUCH SELF TAN CREAM
Best budget buy
£6.59 for 150ml

This moisturizing self-tan delivers a natural-looking colour within three hours. It's available in fair or medium options, to suit most skin tones.

■ NUXE SUBLIMATING GOLDEN DRY OIL
Best bronzing dry oil
£22 for 50ml

Not exactly a fake tan but a dry oil that gives the skin a sun-kissed glow. Enriched with tiny specks of mother of pearl, it is absorbed at once to leave you lustrous.

■ ST TROPEZ AUTO BRONZANT
Best for an all-over glow
£30 for 240ml

This iconic celebrity favourite, once only available in beauty salons, is considered by many to be the ultimate cheat for a deep-bronze glow.

SUN PROTECTORS

■ CLARINS SUN CARE CREAM (SPF 10, 20, 30)
Best suncare range
£16 for 200ml

This water-resistant sunscreen is lightweight and delicately fragranced; it contains a precursor of melanin that aims to boost your tan, while extract of silver birch helps to repair the skin and vanilla moisturizes. The cream is also resistant to water and perspiration, providing long-lasting protection from the sun. Available in a range of SPFs up to 30, which is ideal for children or those with very fair or sun-sensitive skin.

■ **CLARINS SUN WRINKLE CONTROL CREAM FOR FACE (SPF 15)**

Best for the face

£14 for 75ml

A lightweight, non-oily cream, great for even fair skin. Apply every day from spring to late autumn in the northern hemisphere, or year-round in the southern hemisphere.

■ **CLINIQUE CITY BLOCK (SPF 15)**

Best for city living

£12.50 for 40ml

A sheer, oil-free formula, this is a tinted cream that can be worn as foundation or under make-up, giving much-needed protection from UV rays and pollution.

■ **CYCLAX SUN PROTECTION (SPF 2–45)**

Best for sport

£5.99 for 250ml

Non-greasy, and water- and sweat-resistant, this suncare product contains green tea, vitamin E, shea butter and aloe vera – all renowned for their protective and soothing properties – as well as mint and cucumber extracts to cool the skin.

■ **DERMALOGICA SOLAR DEFENSE BOOSTER (SPF 30)**

Best formula to mix with any product

£23.60 for 30ml

This provides broad-spectrum UV protection and can be worn under make-up.

■ **ELEMIS WRINKLE CONTROL SUN SCREEN (SPF 25)**

Best anti-ageing protection

£15.50 for 75ml

This luxurious product feels more like a body lotion than a sun cream. It contains vitamin E and sun filters to shield the skin from harmful sun rays, plus an exotic mixture of coconut, camellia and Tahitian monoi oil to soften and condition the skin, meaning that you tan safely and reduce premature ageing.

■ **GARNIER AMBRE SOLAIRE (SPF 4–60)**

Best light formula with the greatest range of SPFs

from £6

The latest technology gives superb protection against skin-ageing. Now available in ultra-light milk formulas, sprays and creams, and in 15 SPFs from 4 to 60.

■ **HELENA RUBINSTEIN MATT EFFECT SUN PROTECTION (SPF 15)**

Best for a matt finish

£18 for 50ml

If you are someone who dislikes the way that some suncreams give a shiny, greasy look to your skin, then this product is perfect for you. It is a lightweight, non-greasy fluid that has been formulated especially for the face and contains vitamins C and E to give extra protection.

■ LA PRAIRIE SOLEIL SUISSE CELLULAR ANTI-WRINKLE SUN CREAM (SPF 30)

Best for preventing wrinkles

£75 for 50ml

Formulated with La Prairie's renowned energizing and nourishing cellular complex, this high-protection cream not only protects but also moisturizes the skin. It contains powerful antioxidants to guard against free radical damage from the sun, and leaves skin feeling smooth and hydrated.

■ L'OREAL SOLAR EXPERTISE (SPF 25)

Best for the body

£12 for 150ml

A great all-round body product to take on holiday, Solar Expertise offers high protection against burning, skin cancer and premature ageing, while rich moisturizers work to keep skin velvety soft. Its non-greasy texture is easily absorbed by the skin, leaving behind no oily film on the surface.

■ NEAL'S YARD SHEA NUT NATURAL SUNSCREEN (SPF 10)

Best natural suncream

£8.50 for 40g

A rich moisturizing sunscreen is PABA-free and instead uses organic oils and zinc oxide to block damaging UV rays. A blend of shea nut butter, soya oil, sweet almond and lavender to soothe and moisturize the skin as it protects.

■ PIZ BUIN ALLERGY SUN PROTECTION LOTION (SPF 15)

Best for allergy-prone skin

£13.95 for 200ml

An ultra-light, easy-to-absorb lotion that contains extra UVA protection for skin that is prone to sun-induced allergies. It is also free from colour and fragrance, making it ideal for even the most delicate and sensitive skin. Also available in SPF30 for very fair skin or children.

■ PRADA SHIELDING LIP BALM (SPF 15)

Best lip protector

£45 for 30 x 1.5ml

Tinted or non-tinted, this balm protects delicate lip skin from the chapping and cracking that results from sun exposure, with antioxidant vitamin E and panthenol.

■ VICHY CAPITAL SOLEIL EXTREME SUNBLOCK STICK (SPF 25)

Best sunblock stick

£5.50 for 3ml

This sunblock stick is designed to give quick and easy coverage to easily burnt places, such as the nose, ears and eye area. It is ideal for protecting very sensitive skin while sunbathing or skiing, and it can also help prevent cold sores from developing as a result of exposure to the sun.

AFTER SUN

■ THE BODY SHOP ALOE VERA BODY LOTION
Best for moisturizing
£5.50 for 250 ml
This easy-to-use spray uses natural ingredients to cool and hydrate sun-parched skin brilliantly.

■ CLARINS AFTER SUN REPLENISHING MOISTURE CARE
Best for maintaining tan
£21.50 for 50ml
Especially formulated for the face to prolong a tan, this cream contains aloe vera to moisturize, hazelnut oil to nourish, shea butter to regenerate and thyme to refresh.

■ DERMALOGICA AFTER SUN REPAIR
Best for sensitive skin
£22.20 for 104ml
This herb-based treatment balm relieves the classic symptoms of sunburn, such as stinging, redness and irritation. Ingredients include algae and mugwort extracts, cooling cucumber, liquorice root and Japanese alder seed extract to help restore the skin and protect it from further damage.

■ ESTEE LAUDER AFTER SUN REHYDRATING LOTION
Best for normal to oily skin
£16 for 150ml
A light, gentle body moisturizer with aloe vera, this soothes damaged skin and restores moisture, helping to reduce peeling and prolong your tan.

■ GARNIER AMBRE SOLAIRE AFTER SUN SKIN MOISTURIZING SPRAY
Best for cooling and calming
£6.99 for 200ml
This spray, enriched with vitamin E, will soothe and hydrate overexposed skin.

■ LIZ EARLE SUN SHADE BOTANICAL AFTER SUN GEL
Best for all skin types (including sensitive)
£12 for 200ml
Rich in botanical extracts, this soothing gel delivers green tea, aloe vera, cucumber, lavender oil and natural-source vitamin E to calm, cool and nourish.

■ MALIBU SOOTHING AFTER SUN WITH INSECT REPELLENT
Best for tropical holidays
£4.99 for 400ml
A soothing, non-greasy lotion that replenishes natural moisture after sun exposure. It also repels irritating insects for up to four hours, so you can remain unbitten when you go out in the evening.

A long with your hair and clothes, make-up is representative of who you are and what sort of image you are conveying to the rest of the world. It is also the most accessible tool for transformation. Stop and think for a moment – are you still wearing the same lipstick you bought four years ago? Or do you change the brand you buy but never the shade? When was the last time you tried a new way of applying eyeshadow? The truth is that we adhere to the same old make-up routines for most of our lives. After all, it's safer. But taking the time to experiment and to look at new products can inspire you to freshen up your look and keep up-to-date.

Just like fashion, make-up should be fun and can be adapted to suit your mood or the occasion. Selecting the right cosmetics for your skin and tone can involve a little groundwork, but buying products and using them is fairly straightforward (see also pages 24–31). Preparing skin with thorough cleansing and moisturizing, along with choosing compatible textures and colours, will help you to create a flawless, long-lasting finish.

Thanks to new technology, most foundations reflect light brilliantly and give even coverage. Sheer foundation usually contains silicones and imparts a natural look, as do gels. Oil-based foundations are great for dry skins, while cream versions are ideal for older skin as they tend to have a thicker, milky texture. Matt foundation doesn't contain any oil so you must apply it quickly – it dries as soon as it comes into contact with the skin. However, it stays shine-free for a long time, making it good for oily skins. Light-reflecting foundations give a natural-looking 'dewy' complexion, and compact foundations combine the benefits of powder and foundation – but be sure to apply them lightly to avoid a mask-like effect. Tinted moisturizers suit those with smooth, blemish-free complexions or those who are enhancing a tan.

The formulation you choose can create radically different effects, from a subtle wash of colour to a dense, saturated hue. Powders are easy to blend and build up, whereas creams tend to have a more intense pigment. Powder blushers are good for adding translucent colour, while creams are stronger and should be used sparingly. Liquids and gels leave a wash of colour, but can be difficult to blend. Use powder eyeshadows if you want to shade and add definition to the eyes, but choose cream formulas if you want to create intensity. Matt lipsticks have dense colours, tend not to smudge and are long lasting. On the other hand, creamy formulas are more dewy but still strongly coloured, which makes them better for drier lips. Lip glosses impart just a hint of colour and masses of shine, but need frequent application. Ultimately, your skin type and tone will determine what colours and textures look best, and once you're got your foundation right, you can have fun with the rest.

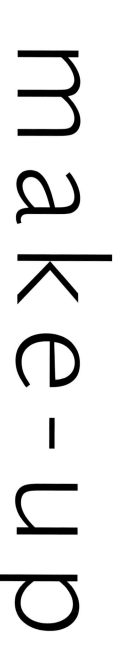

make-up

SKIN BRIGHTENERS

CLARINS BEAUTY FLASH BALM
Best for instant glow
£21.50 for 50ml
Clarins' best-selling product, this herbal balm tightens and brightens even the most tired-looking skin. Used alone or under make-up, it is ideal for concealing the effects of too many late nights.

ESTEE LAUDER SPOTLIGHT SKIN TONE PERFECTOR
Best overall skin brightener
£23 for 50ml
For fresh, luminescent skin, this pearly cream is a must. It contains antioxidants, vitamins C and E and botanicals such as grape and liquorice extract to improve the tone and quality of your skin if used regularly.

LANCOME MAQUISUPERBE
Best skin illuminator
£20 for 30ml
Innovative silicone technology and light-reflective particles give instant luminosity to even the dullest of complexions. Use it neat to highlight your face, or mix it with your foundation. There is gold for warm skin tones and silver for cool skin tones.

MAC STROBE
Best for evenings
£18.50 for 40ml
Mix this ultra-light iridescent cream with your normal foundation, or use it alone to add definition to cheekbones. It contains botanical extracts and vitamins to give skin an instant wake-up call, imparting a natural, healthy glow.

MAKE READY BRIGHTENING MIST
Best spray brightener
£12.50 for 210ml
A superfine spray tones that refines pores and makes skin look brighter. Simply spritz on after cleansing before applying make-up. It can also be reapplied throughout the day to freshen up make-up and tired skin.

PRESCRIPTIVES MAGIC ILLUMINATING LIQUID POTION
Best for giving youthful-looking skin
£25 for 30ml
This pink-tinted iridescent liquid bounces light off imperfections and presents your face in a radiant new light. It perfects the appearance of unevenness and mild discoloration or redness through its revolutionary three-dimensional pigments. Worn over or under foundation, only a tiny amount is needed to leave skin looking fresher and younger.

REVLON SKINLIGHTS FACE ILLUMINATOR (SPF 15)
Best budget skin illuminator
£9.95 for 40ml
A sheer moisturizing liquid, this contains light-refracting minerals such as rose
quartz and mother of pearl to illuminate the skin and give a dewy look. Containing
vitamins C and E, it leaves skin soft and radiant when used alone or mixed with
foundation. Available in four tones: natural, peach, pink and bronze.

ULTIMA II GLOWTION SKIN BRIGHTENING CREAM
Best for dry skin
£20 for 50ml
This unique product creates a veil of shimmering brightness over the skin and
contains vitamins A, C and E to help boost radiance. It is richly moisturizing,
making it perfect for skin that is prone to dryness.

FACE PRIMERS

FRESH FACE PRIMER
Best for dry skin
£24.50 for 30ml
An ultra-light, soothing lotion that prepares the face for make-up application
by filling in fine lines, pores and imperfections to create a smooth surface. It
can also be used as a gentle moisturizer.

LAURA MERCIER FOUNDATION PRIMER
Best for long-lasting make-up
£25 for 44ml
This product acts as a protective layer between your moisturizer and foundation.
Make-up looks fresher, and lasts all day. It contains a refreshing blend of lavender,
orange and rose extracts to tone and pamper skin.

MAKE-UP FOREVER CORRECTIVE MAKE-UP BASE
Best for correcting oiliness
£12.50 for 50ml
A favourite with make-up artists on photo shoots, this oil-free base subtly corrects
skin-tone irregularities, while ensuring foundation is applied evenly. Its mattifying
formula prevents shine from breaking through make-up during the day.

NARS MAKEUP PRIMER
Best for soothing
£22 for 53g
When applied as a base layer, this gel-cream gives foundation a flawless finish. It
contains natural botanicals that reduce redness. Its soothing properties have made
it a favourite post-shave treatment for men, so be sure to hide the tube!

FOUNDATIONS

■ **ALMAY SKIN STAYS CLEAN FOUNDATION**
Best for sensitive skin
£8.99 for 30ml
This lightweight, oil-free formula uses a unique patented betahydroxy complex to help keep out dirt and prevent breakouts. Unlike heavier foundations, this won't clog your skin, but instead allows it to breathe.

■ **AVEDA DUAL BASE MINUS OIL CREAM**
Best for all skin-types
£18 for 9g
A multifunctional, velvety formula, this can be applied with a sponge as a foundation or dry as powder. Rose-scented, with plant-based ingredients, it comes in a recyclable, refillable compact.

■ **BOBBI BROWN FOUNDATION STICK**
Best stick foundation
£26 for 30g
Handily portable, this foundation stick has a highly blendable creamy texture and can also double as a concealer. It comes in 12 of Bobbi's trademark yellow-based shades, which work by adding warmth to the skin.

■ **BOBBI BROWN FRESH GLOW CREAM FOUNDATION**
Best for normal to combination skin
£23 for 30ml
This lightweight, whipped-cream-textured foundation gives medium coverage, and has light-diffusing properties to give a fresh, dewy finish. It contains added vitamins A, C and E and is available in 12 shades.

■ **CHANEL VITALUMIERE SATIN SMOOTHING FLUID MAKE-UP (SPF 15)**
Best for giving youthful-looking skin
£25 for 30ml
The light-reflective properties in this foundation give a flawless, silk-like effect that helps to make the complexion appear softer and more youthful. Its water-in-oil formula glides on effortlessly, while SPF15 and nut extracts provide defence against sun damage.

■ **CHANTECAILLE REAL SKIN**
Best for sheer coverage
£39 for 11g
Almost transparent, this gel-like foundation gives brilliant sheer coverage. A combination of micro-particle powder and oil provides both moisturization and protection against environmental factors. Unbelievably light, it feels almost

as if you are wearing no make-up at all. It is the ideal foundation if you hate the feeling of being 'made up'.

CHANTECAILLE FUTURE SKIN OIL-FREE GEL FOUNDATION
Best for normal to oily skin
£38 for 30g
A water-based, oil-free foundation, this ultra-light formula contains 60 per cent charged water, seaweed extract, green tea, rosemary and rice bran.

CHRISTIAN DIOR TEINT SMOOTHING ANTI-FATIGUE FOUNDATION
Best for tired skin
£21.50 for 30ml
This sheer foundation gives a natural, even finish. It's rich in hydrating ingredients, which moisturize the skin to keep it looking fresh and smooth while also protecting it from environmental damage.

CHRISTIAN DIOR TEINT DIORLIGHT
Best for translucent coverage
£19.50 for 30ml
The translucent, light-reflecting formula bestows a glowing complexion while covering flaws. Being lightweight, it is perfect for summer and the ideal 'in between' if you don't want the heavy coverage of foundation, but find tinted moisturizer too sheer.

CLINIQUE CITYBASE COMPACT FOUNDATION (SPF 15)
Best compact foundation for oily skin
£17.50 for 14g
With special polymers to help this oil-controlling foundation glide on beautifully, it comes in a refillable compact and provides foundation and powder in one. Coverage is easy to control and enduring.

CLINIQUE SUPER-FIT MAKE-UP
Best oil-free everyday foundation
£17 for 30ml
A light, oil-free foundation that delivers excellent coverage, this evens out the tone of the skin without streaking. It lasts all day and won't rub off or wear off with sweat. Skin is left feeling comfortable and looking fresh and matt.

DERMALOGICA TREATMENT FOUNDATION
Best for spot-prone skin
£24.60 for 44ml
Specifically formulated for blemish-prone skin, this gives great coverage while treating the problem. Its oil-free formula contains antioxidant vitamins and natural moisturizers to help protect the skin against environmental assault and moisture loss. Choose from eight shades.

DR HAUSCHKA TRANSLUCENT MAKE-UP
Best organic foundation
£18 for 30ml
An organically based foundation that evens out the complexion and enhances the skin's natural glow. Although light in texture, it gives a flawless finish to the skin. It is ideal for those who prefer chemical-free make-up and is available in three shades.

ERA FACE SPRAY-ON FOUNDATION
Best for a professional finish
£45 for 2.25oz
The application of this innovative spray foundation takes a little time to master, but it's worth it if you want that 'air-brushed' professional finish. It will cover all blemishes and imperfections, while still being light and designed not to cake. Its matt texture means that you don't need to use powder to set your make-up.

ESTEE LAUDER MAXIMUM COVER LIGHTWEIGHT MAKE-UP
Best for full coverage
£19.50 for 30 ml
This waterproof foundation gives full coverage without being at all heavy, and can double as a concealer. Great for wearing during the evening when you need a little more cover.

FASHION FAIR PERFECT FINISH CREAM MAKE-UP
Best for darker skins
£17.50 for 20g
A brilliant soft-finish foundation, this is specifically designed for darker skin tones. It protects skin from external factors such as heat and pollution and is available in seven shades.

GIORGIO ARMANI LUMINOUS SILK FOUNDATION
Best for medium coverage
£25 for 30 ml
A lovely lightweight foundation that hydrates the skin while imparting a silky coverage. Innovative 'micro fil' technology imparts moisture to skin and ensures that the foundation lasts. Almost like a tinted moisturizer, it makes the skin glow and refines the texture. Available in a wide variety of shades.

HELENA RUBINSTEIN ILLUMINATION NATURAL RADIANCE REVIVING MAKE-UP (SPF 15)
Best for oily skins in summer
£25 for 30ml
This oil-free, lightweight formula has light-reflectors to disguise flaws and give skin a wonderful glow. It won't clog pores, stays put all day, and even contains SPF15 to protect skin from the sun.

IMAN SECOND TO NONE OIL-FREE MAKE-UP (SPF 8)
Best oil-free formula for darker skin
£20.95 for 10g

The natural, matt finish is just what darker skins need. Previously this range was aimed at African or Caribbean skin, but now it includes colours that suit all complexions – a clever mixture of neutrals for fair skins and flattering yellow shades for darker ones. Because it is oil-free, it reduces any greasy-looking effect of foundation on darker skins.

LANCOME PHOTOGENIC ULTRA CONFORT (SPF 10)
Best for normal to dry skin
£19.50 for 30ml

A liquid formula that contains moisturizing apricot oil- and light-reflecting pigments, this ensures a flawless finish in any light. Its ability to create perfect-looking skin has made it a bestseller with brides.

LANCOME TEINT IDOLE FOUNDATION
Best for a matt finish
£22.50 for 30ml

Rub-resistant and waterproof to give superb, even coverage for all skin types and to stay put all day. Ideal if you're prone to oiliness, but want to control shine without using a heavy foundation. This fluid foundation is enriched with vitamin E and extracts of white lily and mallow.

LAURA MERCIER OIL-FREE FOUNDATION
Best oil-free formula for a barely there finish
£30 for 30ml

Great for achieving a natural, fresh look, this foundation is peerless. It never feels heavy and gives a barely there finish. It is a particular favourite with make-up artists who need to create skin that looks amazing, even when photographed close up.

LINDA CANTELLO FORGET FOUNDATION (SPF 10)
Best mousse formula
£30 for 30ml

Created by top make-up artist Linda Cantello, this ultra-light mousse formula provides sheer coverage that glides on easily. and is available in four shades. It also contains vitamins C and E to protect and repair your skin.

L'OREAL TRANSLUCIDE HEALTHY GLOW FOUNDATION (SPF 12)
Best budget buy for sheer coverage
£8.99 for 30ml

This lightweight foundation contains light-diffusers and vitamin C, to illuminate skin and diminish the appearance of fine lines and imperfections. It offers high performance at an affordable price.

MAC FACE AND BODY FOUNDATION
Best for face and body
£22 for 120ml
This all-over foundation gives you a porcelain complexion and also works
extremely well on the rest of the body for a seamless finish. Ideal if you are
wearing an outfit that bares the arms and legs.

MAC STUDIO TECH
Best compact foundation for a matt finish
£22 for 50g
A favourite with make-up artists, this all-in-one foundation, concealer and
powder gives a lightweight matt finish. It looks great in natural light, making
it ideal for everyday use.

NEUTROGENA SKIN CLEARING OIL-FREE FOUNDATION
Best budget buy for spot-prone skin
£7.99 for 30ml
Useful for times when skin is blighted by breakouts, this gives medium coverage
with a matt finish. It is non-comedogenic, so it won't clog the skin, and contains
salicylic acid and antibacterial agents to treat spots while it covers them.

PRESCRIPTIVES TRACELESS SKIN-RESPONSIVE TINT
Best for a natural finish
£22 for 30ml
A unique, high-tech tint that gives a totally natural finish that adapts to any light.
It glides on to the skin and camouflages flaws simply by reflecting light off them.

REVLON AGE DEFYING MAKE-UP
Best for mature skin
£11.99 for 37ml
A superhydrating formula, this gives superb, even coverage, smoothing out lines
without caking. Colour particles wrapped in moisturizers hide flaws without
settling into lines. Ideal for slightly older, drier skins that need a richer formulation.

TIPS

- The easiest and quickest way to apply foundation is with a sponge. A wedge-
  shaped one will reach tricky areas, such as the creases around your nose.
- To choose the correct foundation, rub a little on the back of your hand, and
  then wait for five minutes to see if the colour disappears into your skin.
- The best way to cover spots is to apply concealer with a brush. This ensures
  accuracy and allows you to blend colours until the correct shade is achieved.
- After applying foundation, press a tissue against your face to lift off any
  excess – this will help your face to look fresh and natural.

■ REVLON NEW COMPLEXION COMPACT FOUNDATION (SPF 15)
Best long-lasting formula
£9.99 for 37ml
An oil-free, creamy formula, with added sun protection, that is available in 16 shades. It comes with a handy-to-use mirror, making it perfect to carry in your handbag for touch-ups throughout the day.

■ SHU UEMURA NOBARA FOUNDATION
Best for oily skin
£15 for 8g
This compact foundation evens skin tone and provides a satin finish. It also doubles as a concealer and all the shades match with real skin tones. Its formula is ultra-light so it won't clog pores or cause breakouts.

■ TOO FACED BLENDERS
Best for contouring
£20 for 6g
Its stick format makes this double-duty cream-to-powder concealer and foundation easy to blend effortlessly into the skin. Use the lighter shade to disguise imperfections and the darker shade to contour the face.

■ YVES SAINT LAURENT TEINT COMPACT FOUNDATION
Best for dry skin
£29.50 for 10g
Presented in a refillable compact, this foundation rehydrates the facial skin continuously, releasing essential fatty acids throughout the day. Coverage is light, even and amazingly enduring.

TINTED MOISTURIZERS

■ AVEDA MOISTURE PLUS TINT
Best for all skin types
£20 for 50ml
Suitable for all skin types, this gives sheer coverage and provides a little naturally derived SPF protection, plus a lovely rose scent. Ideal if you prefer to use environmentally friendly products.

■ BECCA TINTED GLOW ENHANCER (SPF 26)
Best multifunctional moisturizer
£25 for 50ml
Available in four colours, this multipurpose product offers skincare, make-up and excellent sun protection in one. It possesses hydrating, firming and softening properties, contains vitamins A, B, D and E to increase collagen renewal, and gives a translucent glow.

CLARINS REVITALIZING TINTED MOISTURIZER (SPF 6)
Best for radiance
£19 for 50ml

This provides radiant, fresh coverage for all skin types. Marine algae, sea fennel, mallow and horse chestnut combine to moisturize skin, while vitamins H, B5, C, and E help to protect it from the environment.

ESTEE LAUDER FRESH AIR MOISTURE TINT (SPF 15)
Best for hydrating
£20 for 50ml

The light-as-air formula boasts a time-release delivery system to keep skin superhydrated all day, releasing shea butter, energizing vitamins and bio-mineral water.

VICHY LUMINEUSE
Best for UV protection
£10 for 30ml

A sheer tinted moisturizer that imparts a golden sheen to the face. Hypoallergenic and containing UVA and UVB filters, it is available in two formulas, for dry and normal combination skin, and three shades.

YVES SAINT LAURENT TEINT DE JOUR TINTED MATT MOISTURIZER
Best for a matt finish
£20 for 40ml

Deeply moisturizing and filled with antioxidant ingredients to protect skin from environmental damage, this glides on smoothly to give a sheer, matt finish. Available in six shades.

CONCEALERS

BENEFIT LEMON AID
Best for brighter eyes
£13.50 for 7g

Whether or not you're wearing other make-up, this instant colour corrector will freshen eyelids, brightening the whole eye area in the process. The warm yellow colour eliminates skin discoloration and helps 'lift' the face.

JANE IREDALE CIRCLE/DELETE CONCEALER
Best natural concealer
£23 for 2g

This 100 per cent natural concealer hides under-eye circles impressively. It comes in a useful duo-pack with two shades that can be mixed together to guarantee a perfect finish and contains vitamin K to aid in fading dark circles. It is available in three shades.

LANCOME PALETTE PRO
Best multifunctional concealer
£18 for 1.2ml
There are four creamy shades in this slim compact; beige (to cover flaws), yellow (for under-eye circles), green (to tone down redness) and mauve (to give radiance). The versatility of this product makes it a favourite of make-up artists.

LAURA MERCIER SECRET CAMOUFLAGE
Best for blending
£24 for 7.7g
Providing invisible, convincing coverage for blemishes, the two-shades-in-one compact allow you to blend until you get the colour just right.

MAC SELECT COVER-UP
Best for dry skin
£11 for 15ml
This light, liquid concealer covers imperfections effortlessly. Its comes in a handy tube and its long-lasting formula contains moisturizing ingredients to help skin stay fresh and prevent caking.

MAYBELLINE COVER STICK
Best budget concealer for problem skin
£3.99 for 5ml
Part acne treatment (it contains 0.65 per cent salicylic acid), this aids in the healing of blemishes and won't clog pores while it's covering spots.

ORIGINS QUICK HIDE! EASY BLEND CONCEALER
Best for oily skin
£9 for 7ml
This oil-free concealer blends beautifully to minimize dark circles, wrinkles and redness with its soft-focus diffusers. It also contains soothing cucumber extract.

PAULA DORF EYE LITE
Best concealer for eye area
£19 for 1.6g
A cream that miraculously diffuses light to diminish the prominence of dark circles around the eyes, this gives long-lasting results under foundation while still being subtle enough to use on its own.

PRESCRIPTIVES CAMOUFLAGE CREAM
Best for sensitive skin
£14 for 15ml
A weightless, fragrance-free formula, this has a creamy texture that softens blemishes and under-eye circles. Available in many shades and four skin tone groups, so you can get the perfect match.

YVES SAINT LAURENT RADIANT TOUCH
Best for under-eye circles
£21 for 2.5ml
The ultimate under-eye concealer. Thanks to innovative light-reflecting technology, this brilliant pump-action concealer pen eradicates dark circles and can also be used as a base for eyeshadow or dramatically to diminish the appearance of fine lines.

OIL-BLOTTING SHEETS

ANNA SUI OIL BLOTTING PAPER
Best for scent
£7 for 100 sheets
Lightly scented with rose, these cult papers will freshen your face without disturbing your make-up. Ideal for hot dates.

CLINIQUE STAY MATTE OIL BLOTTING SHEETS
Best for the T-zone
£7.50 for 50 sheets
These come in a dinky pack that will fit discreetly into a micro-bag or even a pocket and will eliminate shine efficiently. Extremely useful in summer or before a job interview when you want to look calm and collected.

MAC BLOT FILM
Best packaging
£10 for 100 sheets
A good size, these sheets also absorb oil brilliantly without drying the skin. So stylish that you won't even mind being seen taking one from your handbag on a night out.

NIVEA VISAGE MATT AND FRESH OIL-ABSORBING AND REFRESHING SHEETS
Best for multipurpose use
£4.95 for 100 sheets
These handy sheets are not only colour-coded but are also dual-action: the green side of the sheet mattifies the skin, while the blue side contains cooling ingredients to refresh it.

SHISEIDO PURENESS OIL-CONTROL BLOTTING PAPER
Best for very oily skin
£12 for 100 sheets
These highly effective sheets not only freshen the skin but also remove shine instantly. This must an essential rescue remedy for skin that is especially prone to oiliness.

LOOSE POWDERS

BOURJOIS LIBRE COMME L'AIR
Best portable powder
£9.95 for 5g
A powder brush with loose powder ingeniously contained in the handle, this is ideal for touch-ups when you're on the move. It delivers the soft, translucent powder evenly over the face for a flawless finish.

CALVIN KLEIN LOOSE POWDER
Best for controlling shine
£18.50 for 9g
Silky fine and oil-free, this powder controls shine and gives a natural finish. It contains light-diffusing silica to soften the appearance of fine lines.

CLINIQUE GENTLE LIGHT POWDER
Best for an iridescent finish
£18.50 for 27g
A glow-giving powder that illuminates the face. The appearance of fine lines are reduced and the skin tone is evened out, thanks to its light-reflecting properties.

CORNSILK ORIGINAL SATIN FACE POWDER
Best for a long-lasting finish
£6.75 for 10g
This classic oil-free powder is made with ground walnut shells rather than talc and helps to fix make-up and control shine without clogging the skin.

ESTEE LAUDER SO INGENIOUS LOOSE POWDER
Best for a flawless finish
£21.50 for 18g
A finely milled powder that glides on to your face, this will finish your make-up perfectly. It comes in three shades and contains specially coated pigments to lock in colour and prevent dryness.

GIORGIO ARMANI LOOSE POWDER
Best for evening glamour
£21.50 for 9g
A fine, translucent powder with a subtle sparkle effect, this is especially good for evening glamour or to enhance bare skin during the day.

PRESCRIPTIVES MAGIC ILLUMINATING POWDER
Best for a luminous finish
£25 for 28g
This innovative powder feels cool on the face as it contains 77 per cent water, which makes it excellent for dry skin or hot days. It diffuses light to give a natural glow.

PRESSED POWDERS

BENEFIT DR FEELGOOD
Best for minimizing visible pores
£19 for 10g
An innovative product that minimizes pores and blots out excess shine. The transparent balm contains vitamins C and E and turns matt when it hits your skin. It can be either patted on top of make-up in place of your normal powder or worn alone for a smooth, velvety finish.

CHANEL DOUBLE PERFECTION COMPACT
Best for a velvet finish
£28 for 15g
Although ultra-sheer, this gives enough coverage to use as a base or over make-up for a powder finish. Apply with a sponge.

FRESH FACE LUSTER
Best for sensitive skin
£36 for 8g
This sheer and hard-to-detect pressed powder can be used either as a light-coverage foundation or as a finishing powder. It delivers a smooth, polished finish to the face without looking caked. Extracts of green tea, aloe and other antioxidants help calm and soothe the skin.

GIVENCHY SEMI-LOOSE FACE POWDER PRISM
Best for blending
£22 for 23g
Each compact contains four shades that blend together to enhance the skin tone naturally and mattify the complexion. Available in five colourways.

HELENA RUBINSTEIN DOUBLE AGENT MATTIFYING PRESSED POWDER
Best for combination skin
£19 for 9g
This unique product has a dual action: it regulates shine on oily areas such as the forehead, nose and chin, but also softens drier zones, such as the cheeks. It contains cucumber extract, renowned for its astringent properties, and white lily extract, an effective moisturizer. Skin is left looking naturally matt.

IMAN LUXURY PRESSED POWDER
Best for dark skin tones
£20.95 for 10g
A fine pressed powder that goes on smoothly and doesn't give a muddy or chalky finish to darker skin, as some non-specialist powders do. It is rich in moisturizers to prevent dryness.

LANCOME HYDRA COMPACT PRESSED POWER
Best for dry skin
£27 for 30g
The powder in this classic and classy black-and-gold compact delivers a luxuriously supersmooth finish and does not cake or clog pores.

RUBY & MILLIE COMPACT POWDER
Best lightweight pressed powder
£16.50 for 6g
This lightweight powder comes in an elegant silver compact. It glides on to the skin for a traceless finish. Available in six shades.

SMASHBOX PHOTO MATTE ANTI-SHINE PRESSED POWDER
Best anti-shine powder
£19 for 15g
Mattifying areas that are prone to shine, brilliantly disguising large pores and creating a more even complexion, this also contains tea tree oil to fight breakouts.

SUGAR POWDERED SUGAR
Best oil-free powder
£12 for 11g
Bestowing a silky, matt finish, this powder is available in three yellow-based tones. (Try the sparkling shimmer powder, too – great for highlighting eyes and cheeks.)

HIGHLIGHTERS

BENEFIT HIGH BEAM
Best for definition
£15 for 15ml
This ingenious product contains subtle pink and gold highlights to add a natural, shimmering glow to the complexion. A dot on the lips or tip of the nose, or a smear on each eyelid, is enough to add shine and definition to your face.

BENEFIT KITTEN
Best all-over shimmer
£19.50 for 10g
Shimmer powder for arms, shoulders, legs and face that is held in a luxurious puff. It comes in three different shades and gives a beautiful sparkle.

THE BODY SHOP GLOW ENHANCER
Best for variety of colours
£10 for 30 ml
A great product that is designed to enhance the skin's natural glow or highlight the contours of the face. Available in four shades: natural, for a subtle fresh-faced

look; copper which imparts a warm glow; gold, for a slight metallic sheen; violet for a cool, illuminated finish. All contain light-reflecting mica pearls, Vitamin E (a well-known antioxidant), panthenol to condition the skin and Marula oil to smooth it. Apply this highlighter before or after foundation, or use alone to add definition to the cheekbones.

COSMETICS A LA CARTE SHINE ON
Best liquid highlighter
£12 for 6ml
A liquid shine product that adds a subtle sparkle to lids, this can also be used on cheekbones and lips. It is non-sticky and comfortable to wear.

EYEKO GLITTER POWDER
Best for evening glamour
£15 for 100g
Choose this all-over body powder with light-reflecting particles to turn pallid skin into sexy, shimmery skin. Gorgeously scented with vanilla, it also comes with a velvety puff.

MAC IRIDESCENT POWDER
Best for a look-at-me glow
£12 for 6g
Use this shimmer powder alone on face or body for a supershiny finish, or mix with moisturizer or foundation for a more dramatic glow.

NARS THE MULTIPLE
Best multipurpose stick
£26 for 14.2g
This creamy stick comes in a range of shades and can be used to add colour and a touch of shimmer to eyes, lips and cheeks – perfect for when you're on the go, it nestles in many a celebrity's bag.

TIPS

- To establish where you should use highlighter, stand under a bright lamp and see where the light falls: if it shines over your cheekbones, for example, this is the area you should highlight.
- For an all-over sheen, mix a little highlighter into your regular foundation before application.
- If you're looking washed out, a stroke of bronzer or blusher across your forehead, where the sun would hit your face, creates a healthy glow.
- To create a natural flushed cheek, never use the brush that comes in a blusher compact – it's too stiff and small. Instead, invest in a good blusher brush that is at least 5 cm (2 in) in diameter.

PASSPORT NOMAD ANYWHERE COLOUR
Best oil-free stick
£12.50 for 3.4g
From the makers of the portable make-up line Passport comes this lightweight cream colour stick. Use it on eyes and lips or to highlight the cheeks. It's oil-free and enriched with vitamins A, C and E.

ROCKET CITY STAR DUST
Best shimmer for decolletage and shoulders
£11 for 50g
This body shimmer imparts real sparkle when worn on areas such as the shoulders or decollétage. Dust on for seductively glistening skin, gently scented with vanilla.

STILA ALL OVER SHIMMER POWDER
Best powder highlighter
£24 for 8.5g
For an effortlessly glamorous glow, Stila's all over shimmer imparts a subtle, warm look to the face with just a hint of sparkle. Ideal for highlighting eyes or the collarbones or accentuating cheekbones. Also available in a lightweight, fragrance-free cream formula for the body.

BRONZERS

BLOOM ALOHA BRONZER
Best for a light glow
£18.95 for 15g
Scented with lavender essential oil and containing a light sunscreen, this glides on to create a healthy glow in a flash, without clogging pores. It comes in a handy compact with mirror.

BOBBI BROWN BRONZING POWDER
Best for a smooth finish
£30 for 8g
Formulated for all skin types in believable tan colours, this lightweight, fragrance-free powder with vitamin E goes on smoothly and evenly. A natural, sun-kissed look is the result.

CARGO BRONZER
Best for iridescence
£18 for 8g
Developed with the consultation of some of the world's leading make-up artists, this illuminating, fine powder gives cheeks an iridescent glow either to extend an already existing tan or to add life to a pale winter complexion. Choose from three shades: light, medium or dark.

CHANEL BRONZE UNIVERSEL
Best sheer bronzer
£20 for 24g
For a St Tropez complexion, invest in this incredibly easy-to-use cream-to-powder bronzer. Simply blend it over cheeks for an ultra-sheer glow, or use all over the face on top of moisturizer for a more intense effect.

CLARINS BRONZING DUO
Best for all skin tones
£21 for 11g
This lightweight compact powder imparts a light glow with mother of pearl to reflect light. It is available in two shades – Morning Sun for fair skin and Bright Sun for darker skin.

CLINIQUE BRUSH-ON SUN OIL-FREE POWDER
Best for a matt finish
£15.50 for 10g
Apply this directly to bare skin or over foundation to transform winter pallor to summer colour in a matter of seconds. It's oil-free so it won't clog pores or leave skin looking shiny, and the effect lasts all day.

ESTEE LAUDER INSTANT SUN DUO-TONE BRONZER
Best for face and decolletage
£20 for 14.4g
Containing both vitamin E and ceramides to hydrate the skin, this powder bronzer delivers a convincing sun-kissed glow while preventing shine. Use the lighter side to achieve an all-over glow and the darker side on cheekbones.

GUERLAIN TERRACOTTA BRONZING POWDER
Best for natural sparkle
£22 for 10g
Very natural-looking, this bronzer contains just a hint of sparkle to liven it up. Available in four shades, it offers some sun protection and gives a fabulous glow.

LANCOME STAR BRONZER (SPF 8)
Best bronzing pen
£25 for 5g
When clicked, this clever powder-brush pen delivers a luminous line of bronzing powder onto the face and body. Very handy for beach holidays or when travelling.

LAURA MERCIER BRONZING POWDER
Best two-tone bronzer
£24 for 8.1g
This bronzer can be worn over foundation or alone to add a subtle glow to the skin. Blend the two powders to create your perfect shade.

PRESCRIPTIVES BRONZING POWDER
Best for a natural look
£20 for 8g
In a dual-sided compact, this gives a very natural-looking glow to the skin. It's lightweight and long-lasting, with a versatile matt or pearly finish, so you can alternate as the mood takes you.

PRETTY PRETTY FACE LITE
Best for shading
£22 for 7g
This compact contains two cream-to-powder colours to add a golden bronze to the face. Ideal for shading, highlighting or adding shape, it is enriched with vitamins A and E to moisturize and protect and contains natural sun filters.

REVLON NEW COMPLEXION BRONZING POWDER
Best oil-free budget buy
£8.29 for 8g
An oil-free powder that creates a sheer bronze radiance that really lasts. Its silky, light formula makes it easy to blend and long lasting. As it's fragrance-free, it's suitable for sensitive skin.

STILA SPORT COLOR PUSH-UP IN BRONZE FLASH
Best bronzing stick
£14 for 9g
This handy bronzing stick gives instant fresh, sheer colour. A multipurpose product, it can be used on the face for an all-over sheen or just on cheeks and lips. The gel-based formula hydrates skin, while acting as a protective barrier against the elements.

POWDER BLUSHERS

CHANEL JOUES CONTRASTE
Best for iridescence
£24.50 for 5g
Slightly iridescent, this powder blusher has a light texture and comes in a sleek black compact. Its silky formula makes for easy application and subtle blending.

CHRISTIAN DIOR BLUSH
Best for a soft finish
£21.50 for 3.5g
This fabulous soft powder blush can be used to highlight, accent and sculpt the cheekbones. Ultra-light talc and mica particles coated in amino acids deliver an extra-fine finish for a flawless, natural look that brings a flush of colour to the cheeks. It is available in six shades.

GIORGIO ARMANI SHEER BLUSH
Best for layering
£19 for 7.5g
A powder blusher that blends easily into the skin to produce a sheer, tinted glow. Thanks to the wonder of micro-fill technology, it can then be layered to achieve a more intense colour yet still avoid caking. Available in five shades, it also comes in a fluid version.

GIVENCHY POWDER BLUSH
Best for versatility
£21 for 12g
This compact gives you a choice between matt and subtly shimmery so you can choose between the two or blend them for a luminescent glow. It blends well into the apples of the cheeks and won't brush off.

JOEY NEW YORK CHISELED CHEEKS
Best for shading
£16 for 3g
Specifically designed to give the impression of higher cheekbones, this innovative blush set comes with three specially formulated and coloured blushes: Definition, a powder blush to be applied under the cheekbones; Glow, a powder blush to be applied on the apples of the cheeks; and Accent, a cream blush to be applied on the higher cheek area.

MAC MATTE POWDER BLUSH
Best for oily skin
£12 for 6g
A pressed powder blush that blends easily and stays put throughout the day. Comprised of matt-finish particles and pigments which reflect colour, it gives skin a flawless finish and prevents shine breakthrough. Choose from more than 39 fabulous shades.

NARS BLUSH
Best lasting blush
£16.50 for 4.5g
Designed to naturally highlight the complexion, it has a great easy-to-blend formula. There are 14 enticing shades, including the make-up artists' favourite, Orgasm, a slightly shimmery peachy-pink.

SHE SHE GET CHEEKY BLUSH
Best for a fresh look
£5 for 5g
From the flirty, fun cosmetic line comes this sheer, natural-finish blush. Add a fresh flush to the face with this intensely pigmented, long-lasting shades. Dust it lightly over the cheekbones for a youthful rosiness.

CREAM, GEL AND LIQUID BLUSHERS

■ **BECCA CREAM BLUSH**
Best for travel
£15 for 3g
This creamy blusher blends wonderfully into the skin and comes in a tiny compact, making it a handbag essential to create radiance on the go.

■ **BENEFIT BENETINT**
Best for lips and cheeks
£21.50 for 50ml
Apply a small amount of this beauty editors' favourite liquid tint with a make-up sponge or fingers and blend out gently. It can be used on lips as well as cheeks for an innocent yet provocative flush and is suitable for all complexions.

■ **BENEFIT CHEEKIES**
Best for dry skin
£16 for 14g
A cream blusher that comes in a 1950s-style tube with a sponge applicator. The four pretty shades all give skin an almost translucent glow.

■ **BLOOM SHEER COLOUR CREAM**
Best for cheeks and eyes
£11.50 for 5g
This cream blusher from the cult Australian range imparts shimmery highlights to cheeks and eyes as well. Available in a range of dewy colours, it is perfect for creating that virtuous 'just left the gym' flush.

■ **CLINIQUE BLUSH WEAR**
Best for a subtle glow
£12.50 for 5g
An easily blendable cream-to-powder blusher, this glides on easily when applied with fingers and gives a subtle glow. It stays put all day.

■ **HELENA RUBINSTEIN LIQUID COLOUR BLUSHER**
Best long-lasting liquid blusher
£20 for 20ml
These wearable colours give the cheeks a natural glow and last well throughout the day. The liquid formula makes it easy to blend for a light finish.

■ **LANCOME BLUSH FOCUS**
Best everyday blusher
£12.50 for 2.5g
This cream-to-powder blusher gives a natural-looking outdoorsy flush and comes in a marvellous variety of colours. An everyday necessity.

ORIGINS PINCH YOUR CHEEKS
Best for a natural look
£9 for 3ml
Squeeze from the tube and use the tiniest dab of these berry-coloured gels over moisturizer for a glowing, fresh finish. Ideal for adding light colour to cheeks over the winter months.

PIXI NATURAL CHEEK GEL
Best alternative to blusher
£14 for 14g
Created by three Swedish sisters whose products testify to their motto, 'I just want to look as though I've had a good night's sleep', this is a lighter alternative to blusher. The easy-to-apply transparent cream-gel comes in three natural shades to suit any skin tone.

RUBY & MILLIE FACE GLOSS
Best for a non-greasy glow
£12 for 10g
This multipurpose stick gives a non-greasy sheen to cheeks, lips and eyes. Use on bare skin or over foundation for a subtle, ultra-modern glow.

STILA CONVERTIBLE COLOUR
Best for soft, creamy texture
£23 for 4.25g
A soft cream blusher in a pretty compact that delivers a natural glow to the cheeks and can also be used on the lips. It is long-lasting and great for highlighting. Blend it over your foundation for the best effect.

EYESHADOW BASES

DELUX BEAUTY MULTIPURPOSE PRIMER
Best for priming eyes and lips
£18 for 9g
Created by Hollywood make-up artist Jillian Dempsey, this lightweight, dual-purpose primer can be patted onto lids to prevent eyeshadow from creasing or dabbed on lips to prevent lipstick from feathering. It is invisible, so you can then apply colour on top, as normal.

ESTEE LAUDER LUCIDITY LIGHT-DIFFUSING CONCEALER (SPF 8)
Best for disguising flaws
£15 for 2ml
Its light-diffusing properties camouflage pigmentation and tiny veins, while camomile, aloe vera and cucumber soothe the eyes, it also helps to keep eyeshadow in place all day.

COSMETICS A LA CARTE SECRET LIGHT
Best light-reflecting eye base
£17 for 8g
Light-reflecting pigments help to diffuse light away from dark shadows, redness and fine lines, while volatile silicones help this hardworking eye base glide on. Available in eight shades.

ORIGINS UNDERWEAR FOR LIDS
Best for holding colour in place
£10 for 1.8g
These flesh-coloured, slightly shimmery lid bases help stop eyeshadow from creasing. They also contain gentle moisturizers to care for the delicate skin around the eyes. Ideal for mature skin.

POWDER EYESHADOWS

BENEFIT ISLAND HOT SPOTS
Best iridescent eyeshadow
£13.50 for 1.7g
A seriously sexy iridescent eyeshadow to add instant sparkle to eyes, this comes in three different shades, each in a dinky mirrored compact.

BOBBI BROWN EYESHADOW
Best matt eyeshadow
£13.50 for 1.7g
This densely pigmented eyeshadow contains special polymers for long-lasting colour, and comes in a wide range of subtle, wearable shades with a matt finish. Safe for contact lens wearers.

BOURJOIS SUIVEZ MON REGARD
Best shimmering loose eyeshadow
£6.50 for 1.5g
If you want supershine, glamorous colour intensity and an iridescent finish, this the product for you. Use it as a gentle colour wash over the lids during the day or as an extra highlight for a dramatic night-time look. Choose from 10 sparkling shades for luminous lids. Each comes in a handy pot with a brush so the shadow won't spill everywhere.

CHANEL LES 4 OMBRES EYESHADOW
Best for up-to-the-minute colours
£30.50 for 4g
These gorgeous eyeshadow quartets give deep, long-lasting colour with a luminous finish. Shades are coordinated and can be used dry for a subtle effect, or wet for more intense colour.

CHANTECAILLE LASTING EYESHADOW
Best non-crease formula
£16.50 for 2.5g
You can apply this ultra-fine eyeshadow colour either wet or dry, depending on the look you want to create. It adheres well to the lid and the colour stays true without creasing. It is packed full of ginseng to condition the skin and comes packaged in a handy single compact.

CHRISTIAN DIOR 5-COLOUR EYESHADOW
Best for mixing colours
£29 for 2.4g
Five silky smooth powder eyeshadows are combined in a covetable compact. The subtle colours are updated seasonally and are created to gently blend and complement each other.

CLE DE PEAU BEAUTE OMBRE COULEUR
Best for delicate skin
£10 for 2.5g
Available in a vast selection of fashionable colours, these eyeshadows don't crease and glide effortlessly across lids. Perfect for delicate skin.

ESTEE LAUDER PURE COLOUR EYESHADOW
Best for fine texture
£13.50 for 1.7g
With an enormous range of up-to-the-minute shades, these silky eyeshadows are cleverly packaged in clear cubes, complete with a mirror and applicator.

GIRL COSMETICS VELVET EYESHADOW
Best for young skin
£12 for 1.7g
Available in a huge variety of fun, look-at-me shades, this eyeshadow smooths over lids effortlessly and blends naturally.

HARD CANDY EYESHADOW COMPACT QUARTET
Best lasting eyeshadow
£28.95 for 7.9g
These glamorous matt and sparkling eyeshadow quartets go on smoothly and won't disappear by lunchtime. They come with a sponge applicator for blending and an angled brush for lining eyes.

L'OREAL COLOUR APPEAL EYESHADOW
Best budget buy
£4.99 for 1.7g
This product delivers good texture at an accessible price, and is available in a good range of colours, from the natural to the dramatic.

MAC EYESHADOW
Best for a glittery finish
£9 for 1.5g
Either apply this sexily shimmering eyeshadow on its own to lids, or use sparingly to enhance matt eyeshadows. A favourite among models and make-up artists around the world.

PHYSICIAN'S FORMULA PEARLS OF PERFECTION
Best for sensitive skin
£6 for 1.7g
A product line formulated specifically for the needs of sensitive skin, this eyeshadow is hypoallergenic and fragrance free. The matt and shimmery multicoloured eyeshadow pearls combine to illuminate eyes and give a subtle shimmer to the lids.

POOLE SEPARATES EYE COLOUR
Best for a velvet finish
£12 for 1.9g
Highly pigmented, this silky powder doesn't crease. Use dry for a velvety effect, or wet for more definition.

PUPA EXTRALIGHT EYESHADOW DUO
Best for a luminous sheen
£11.95 for 1.6g
Using innovative tiny pearls to give sparkle, this extremely light textured eyeshadow not only adds a luminous sheen to lids, but also has excellent staying power so that your eyes will shimmer all night long.

SHU UEMURA PRESSED EYESHADOW
Best for a metallic finish
£12.50 for 2.8g
These silky shadows are available in an incredible variety of natural and dramatic colours and in matt, iridescent, metallic and pearl finishes. The shades work beautifully together and can create a perfect evening look.

TIPS

- Apply a light covering of concealer over your eyelids to even out skin tone, hide redness and help to make your eyeshadow stay put for longer.
- If your eyes are deep-set, apply a light shade to the eyelid and a medium, neutral colour to the brow bone. This will give eyes a more balanced and brighter look.
- To make a shade of powder eyeshadow more intense and vibrant, simply moisten the brush before you dip it in the eyeshadow.

CREAM AND GEL EYESHADOWS

BOURJOIS EFFET DE NACRE
Best for smoky eyes
£5.75 for 10ml
Perfect for creating a sexy, smudged look, this easy-to-blend cream eyeshadow range gives a crease-free and hardwearing finish. There's a wide range of shades.

CLINIQUE TOUCH TINT FOR EYES
Best subtle cream eyeshadow
£12 for 7ml
This water-based cream-to-powder shadow has a slight shimmer, is long-lasting and available in seven shades. It gives a subtle creaseproof glow to eyes.

GUERLAIN DIVINORA CREAM-TO-POWDER EYESHADOW
Best for a smooth finish
£13 for 1.5g
Available in six shades, these glide on incredibly smoothly and do not crease or fade. The exquisite hammered-gold pot is irresistible.

LANCOME COLOUR FOCUS CREME
Best for dry skin
£13 for 12ml
Richly moisturizing, this eye colour goes on smoothly and provides maximum comfort throughout the day – even on dry skin. The great range of funky colours gives you plenty of scope to experiment.

LINDA CANTELLO CREAM EYESHADOW
Best for translucent colour
£14.50 for 14g
Supersubtle, this cream eyeshadow in luscious shades glides effortlessly across the lids for lasting, weightless colour that stays true without fading.

MAC EYE GLASS
Best for shine
£15 for 2.5g
A clear gloss, this product can be worn alone or mixed with cream eyeshadow to create a very contemporary look. It contains an emollient for comfort and vitamin E.

MAYBELLINE COOL EFFECTS EYE COLOUR TUBE
Best for summer
£3.99 for 8ml
This eye cream, which lasts up to eight hours, glides on to lids with a fresh, cooling sensation. The effect is light and shimmery, but not greasy. It can be used on lips and cheeks, too. Try blending shades to make your perfect colour.

RUBY & MILLIE EYE COLOUR CREAM
Best for easy application
£12 for 8ml
Smooth, creamy eyeshadows contained in a stylish pen applicator, which you
simply twist to release colour directly on to your lids. They are easy to blend and
long lasting. For a less intense effect, apply the colour close to the lash line and fill
in the rest of the lid with a slightly lighter shade.

PENCIL EYELINERS

BARRY M GLITTER EYE CRAYON
Best sparkling eyeliner
£4.50 for 1.1g
Fine particles in this glitzy product give a smooth, powdery application, adding a
sexy sparkle to come-hither eyes. Available in blue, pink, lilac, white and silver, it
makes a great highlighter for shimmering evening eyes.

CHANEL PRECISION EYE DEFINER
Best creamy eyeliner
£14 for 2.5ml
A very creamy formula, neither hard nor waxy, this comes with a built-in blender
sponge. Choose between a clear, precise line around the eye or a gentle shadow
beneath. Safe for contact lens wearers.

CHRISTIAN DIOR EYE LINER PENCIL
Best for definition
£11 for 1.2g
Comes with a blending tip and sharpener for marvellous matt definition. Ideal for
precise lining, but with a soft easy-to-apply texture. Use the foam tip for softening
lines or alternatively to blend in eyeshadows.

ELIZABETH ARDEN SMOKY EYES POWDER PENCIL
Best for blending
£12 for 1.1g
The smooth, creamy formula makes this a liner and shadow in one. It gives
striking definition and can be used to create sultry eyes when smudged with
the applicator tip.

LAURA MERCIER EYE LINER
Best long-lasting eyeliner
£12.50 for 1.2g
A cake eye liner that stays put and gives great definition, it can also be softened by
using it with a damp eye liner brush. It comes in a good range of natural-looking
shades that match skin and eye tones.

LORAC CREAM EYELINER COLLECTION
Best for a smudgy finish
£25 for 6g
Choose from eight creamy colours (gold, black, copper, silver, grey, brown, purple and charcoal) to accent and define eyes. Smudge it on dry for a soft, sexy look, or apply wet for intense definition; there is a double-sided brush in the compact.

NARS EYE LINER PENCIL
Best for sensitive eyes
£12.50 for 1.2g
Dermatologist-tested and fragrance-free, this has intense pigments to give a rich, velvety look. Lines can be left precise or smudged to achieve a smoky effect.

TONY AND TINA HERBAL GLITTER PENCIL
Best for a glittery finish
£12.50 for 1.4g
A supersoft eyeliner that adds a touch of sparkle to eyes, it contains chickweed to help fight irritation, chamomile to soothe, cucumber to firm and aloe to moisturize.

LIQUID EYELINERS

GIVENCHY DEFINITION FLUID EYELINER MIROIR
Best for strong definition
£16 for 1.2ml
This automatic, click-action pen guarantees a precise line. The softly tapered brush deposits just the right amount of colour to give eyes deep, lasting definition.

INKLINGS LIQUID EYE LINER
Best for intense colour
£12 for 2.2g
One simple stroke from this long-lasting eyeliner will impart an intense colour. The finish is smooth and feels comfortable on the skin.

LANCOME ARTLINER
Best for easy use
£17.50 for 1.4ml
This eyeliner comes with a 'felt-tip' applicator enabling even beginners and those with wobbly hands to create a line at the edge of the lashes in a single stroke.

MAKE-UP FOR EVER COLOUR LINER
Best long-lasting liquid eyeliner
£8.75 for 4ml
Intense colours with outstanding durability, these are unbeatable for a striking evening look. Suitable for contact lens wearers or those with skin allergies.

NARS LIQUID EYELINER
Best for fine lines
£22 for 7ml
This liquid liner comes complete with an ultra-thin lining brush, to paint a fine and precise sliver of colour either on top of or under lids. Available in 12 jewel-inspired tones that last all day and all night.

SHISEIDO LIQUID EYE LINER
Best waterproof eyeliner
£16 for 6ml
With a diamond-shaped brush for easy application, this eyeliner is waterproof so it's just the thing for April showers or 'weepies' at the cinema. It is available in a wide range of natural-looking shades.

TARTE DOUBLE-ENDED EYE LINER
Best for sexy eyes
£12 for 1.9g
This creamy pencil is your weapon if you want sexy, smudgy eyes. Double-ended, it has a black pencil at one end and your choice of plum, khaki, navy or brown at the other.

BOBBI BROWN LONG-WEAR GEL EYE LINER
Best for dramatic eyes
£13.50 for 31g
The highly pigmented gel formula provides the precision of liquid eye liner. Dip the tip of the supplied brush into the pot and coat both sides, removing any excess, before applying. You will need to work fast as it dries quickly.

MASCARA

CHANEL DRAMA LASH EXTREME WEAR MASCARA
Best for separating
£15 for 8ml
This heavy, creamy formula coats lashes without clumping and contains pro-vitamin B5 and ceramides to condition. The ingenious two-zone brush has different-shaped bristles to add volume and separate at the same time.

CHRISTIAN DIOR FASCINATION FREE STYLE ENHANCING MASCARA
Best for curling
£15 for 7ml
Choose this curling mascara for extra lift. For stunning results, use the wand to pull up lashes, and hold for six seconds. It creates a catwalk effect and won't clump or flake.

CLARINS PURE VOLUME MASCARA
Best for everyday wear
£15.50 for 7ml
Based on vegetable waxes, this has a creamy texture and leaves lashes glossier, more supple and enviably defined. It stays put all day and all night.

CLINIQUE LASH DOUBLING MASCARA
Best for volumizing
£12 for 8g
Add both volume and extra length to lashes with this impressive product. The precision brush means every lash is coated evenly without becoming clogged.

DR HAUSCHKA MASCARA
Best natural mascara
£14 for 8ml
Made of entirely natural ingredients such as black tea extract, lightly scented with rose and incredibly easy to remove at night, this is great for everyday use.

ESTEE LAUDER ILLUSIONIST MAXIMUM CURLING MASCARA
Best for lifting
£15.50 for 7ml
This innovative mascara uses revolutionary aerospace and textile technology to deliver a dramatic lift and curl to lashes, to really open up the eyes. Air-gel spheres create maximum volume without weight for an effect that lasts all day, and the high-tech brush is twice as wide and twice as thick as traditional brushes.

GUERLAIN DIVINORA ENTICING EYES MASCARA
Best for curling and volumizing
£14.50 for 8ml
This mascara contains wheat to plump up sparse lashes. Its unique brush design enhances volume and curls lashes by more than 36 per cent. Lashes look noticeably fuller and the colour won't smudge off during the day.

TIPS

- To apply liquid eyeliner precisely, try drawing three dashes – one at the inside corner, one in the middle of the lash line and another at the outer corner. Then simply go back and join up the dashes.
- Keep a cotton bud handy, soaked in eye make-up remover, to clean up eyeliner or mascara mistakes without smearing the rest of your make-up.
- Always curl your lashes before applying mascara or you will risk damaging the lashes. Gently heating a metal lash curler with a hairdryer will help set the curl.
- For professional, clump-free lashes, always separate the lashes after applying your mascara, using an eyelash comb.

HELENA RUBINSTEIN EXTRAVAGANT MASCARA
Best non-smudge mascara
£17 for 7ml
This fantastic smudge-proof, clump-proof formula gives a seriously even, refined look. Best of all, it doesn't leave behind any telltale flakes under the eyes.

KISS ME MASCARA
Best black mascara
£16.50 for 4.5g
A Japanese favourite, apply this and leave to set for two minutes to create long, lush lashes. The smudge-proof formula is gentle enough for sensitive eyes.

LANCOME DEFINICILS
Best thickening mascara
£16 for 6.5ml
The unique brush design enables the mascara to glide smoothly on to lashes in a fine, even layer while the innovative formula coats them, particularly at the tips, without forming clumps.

LANCOME ETERNICILS MASCARA
Best for a flawless finish
£16 for 6.5ml
This 100 per cent waterproof mascara will last through swimming or workouts without smudging. It has micro-curled latex, which unrolls on contact with lashes, giving great definition. Lashes are coated one by one, resulting in a smooth finish.

L'OREAL LONGITUDE WATERPROOF MASCARA
Best lengthening budget mascara
£17.99 for 7ml
The high-definition brush increases the separation of lashes, while L'Oreal's Extensel formula lengthens lashes by more than 30 per cent.

MAC PRO LASH MASCARA
Best for sensitive eyes
£8 for 7.5g
The best long-lasting mascara for naturally full-looking lashes, this hardworking, professional formula lengthens, thickens and defines without smudging. Make-up artists highly rate its great depth of colour. It is fragrance free and hypoallergenic.

MAX FACTOR 2000 CALORIE MASCARA
Best for contact lens wearers
£7 for 9ml
Fragrance-free and hypoallergenic, this touch-proof and rub-proof formula is able to resist heat, moisture and abrasion. The refined brush delivers just the right amount of mascara to lashes to create a thick, glossy, clump-free finish.

MAYBELLINE GREAT LASH MASCARA
Best budget mascara
£4.49 for 12.5ml

This is the world's most famous and bestselling mascara, proved by the fact that, around the world, one is sold every 1.9 seconds. A particular favourite of make-up artists in film and television, it colours and separates lashes brilliantly for a gentle, natural look.

MAYBELLINE LASH DISCOVERY ONE BY ONE WATERPROOF MASCARA
Best waterproof mascara
£6.49 for 5ml

The mini brush separates each lash individually as the mascara is applied, so it covers even the hard-to-reach corner lashes, while advanced polymer technology ensures that there is no clumping.

ORIGINS FRINGE BENEFITS MASCARA
Best for conditioning
£9 for 6ml

Lash-conditioning ingredients include Damascene rose, carnuba wax and camomile, enriching a formula that glides on smoothly, giving natural definition and length to lashes.

REVLON COLORSTAY EXTRA THICK LASHES MASCARA
Best volumizing budget mascara
£7.99 for 8ml

This heavy, thick mascara does build the most amazing volume but you may need to use a lash comb for separating lashes afterwards. Especially good for a dramatic evening effect.

SISLEY DOUBLE ACTION PHYTO MASCARA
Best for strengthening
£21 for 8g

This not only gives maximum volume, and also lengthens lashes. The brush is made of strong natural-silk fibres and separates lashes one by one, while the creamy yet light formula with pro-vitamin B5, soya extract and gardenia flower extract strengthens them.

YVES SAINT LAURENT FALSE LASH EFFECT MASCARA
Best for a flawless finish
£17 for 7.5ml

Made up of a concoction of nylon, polymers, waxes, pro-vitamin B5, brown seaweed gel and aloe, this ultra-glamorous mascara builds incredible length and volume with a superflawless finish. It is gentle enough for sensitive eyes and contact lens wearers.

EYEBROW COLOURS

THE BODY SHOP BROW AND LASH TINT
Best for keeping eyebrows neat
£7 for 7ml
Containing vitamins and plant extracts, this clear gel not only ensures that brows stay in shape but also in good condition. It can be used as an alternative to mascara for a more relaxed, natural look.

BRENDA CHRISTIAN UNIVERSAL BROW DEFINER PENCIL
Best for a natural look
£11.50 for 8g
An ingenious pencil that looks grey but amazingly it works with the skin's pH to create a colour that is identical to your hair colour – irrespective of whether you are blonde, jet black or red! The perfect accessory for creating natural-coloured eyebrows easily.

CHANEL PERFECT BROWS
Best eyebrow kit
£29 for 5g
This compact really has everything you might need for achieving perfect eyebrow arches. The elegant compact includes three eyebrow powders, which could also double as eyeliners, a pair of tweezers, a brow-defining brush and even a magnifying mirror.

CHRISTIAN DIOR POWDER BROW PENCIL
Best for groomed eyebrows
£11 for 7g
This soft pencil comes in a range of natural-looking colours, and includes its own brush for combing your eyebrows into shape. Ideal for those who want to achieve a clean, groomed look. Essentially, it is equipped with a good-quality pencil sharpener.

TRUCCO HIGH BROW TRIO
Best for defining brows
£30 for 6g
A compact containing three complementary shades, so you can get a perfect colour match for your eyebrows.

VINCENT LONGO BRUSH ON BROW
Best for arched brows
£14 for 4g
Arch and define brows in a matter of seconds with a choice of four natural-looking shades. Currently very popular with New York make-up artists, who love the professional finish it creates.

LIP PRIMERS

BENEFIT DEGROOVIE
Best for use in hot weather
£18 for 6g
An invisible barrier that prevents your lipstick moving anywhere – even on a hot, sunny day! The soft, clear wax melts into the fine creases around the lips so lipstick has an invisible boundary and lines are softened.

BENEFIT LIP PLUMP
Best for a full pout
£13.50 for 10ml
This lip plump is a blend of jojoba oil and waxes with flesh-toned pigments. It has the effect of building up and dramatically enhancing the contours of the mouth, giving the impression of sensationally full, pouty lips. A truly miraculous foundation for lips.

ESTEE LAUDER LIPZONE ANTI-FEATHERING COMPLEX
Best for mature skin
£17.50 for 15ml
A lightweight gel-creme that moisturizes and softens lips, thus reducing the appearance of fine lines and helping to eliminate lipstick feathering. For best results apply the product before your lipstick, smoothing onto the area just outside the natural lip line.

MAKE UNDER LIP SLEEK
Best for preventing flaking
£10 for 4g
This clear balm smoothes and moisturizes lips, making lipstick glide on more easily, look fresher and last for longer without flaking or becoming dry. It comes with its own mini lip brush for easy application.

SCREENFACE LIP PRIMER
Best for a professional finish
£7.50 for 6.25g
A light cream that comes with an easy-to-use applicator wand and will help your lipstick to last all day long. It is rich in natural moisturizers, which work to nourish and smooth the lips so that lipstick glides on more easily thus creating a superb, flawless finish.

SMASHBOX LID AND LIP PRIMER
Best for preventing colour fade
£19 for 25g
This dual-use wonder product dares any lipstick or eyeshadow to fade, bleed, or crease before its time. Apply to cleansed lips and eyelids before make-up.

LIP LINERS

BENEFIT SILK LIP SKETCHING PENCIL
Best for a natural look
£12.50 for 2.1g
A super-soft lip pencil that blends into the lip line for natural-looking definition. Its extra soft and sponge-tipped for easy blending, helping create the perfect pout.

CHANEL PRECISION LIP DEFINER
Best for definition
£14.50 for 1g
This creamy-textured pencil has silicones for ease of application, and comes with its own brush for precise definition. It also contains vitamin E to moisturize and protect lips.

CLINIQUE QUICK LINER
Best water-resistant lip liner
£11 for 0.3g
This is a propelling pencil so it needs no sharpening. It glides on smoothly as you draw so lipstick doesn't feather, and it's water-resistant and fragrance-free.

ELIZABETH ARDEN LIP DEFINER PENCIL
Best colour range
£8.50 for 0.25g
A propelling pencil with impressive staying power, available in a vast number of shades. It also contains conditioning ingredients to hydrate lips and help prevent colour fade.

LAURA MERCIER LIP PENCIL
Best for preventing feathering
£9 for 1.4g
A moisturizing lip pencil that gives superb definition and helps to prevent lipstick feathering, making it excellent for mature skins.

MAC LIP PENCIL IN 'SPICE'
Best natural colour
£9 for 1.4g
A perennial favourite of celebrities and make-up artists, this is as close as you can get to your natural lip colour and genuinely stays put.

ORIGINS LIP PENCIL
Best lasting liner
£8.50 for 1.2g
Featherproof, waterproof and incredibly long-lasting, this provides great definition. Ideal for wearing in hot climates or while playing sport.

LIPSTICKS

CHANEL HYDRABASE
Best for up-to-the-minute colours
£13.50 for 3.5g
This is soft and easy to wear and won't smudge. Its rich formula glides on easily and contains SPF15 to protect against UV damage.

CLARINS LE ROUGE
Best hydrating lipstick
£13 for 3.5g
A lightly scented lipstick that provides non-budge, long-lasting colour, while hydrating the lips with ingredients such as wheatgerm oil, shea butter and vitamins C and E.

ELIZABETH ARDEN EXCEPTIONAL LIPSTICK
Best non-feathering lipstick
£12.50 for 4g
Moisturizing ceramides produce a creamy formula with super staying power that lives up to its name. It is available in eight classic shades.

ESTEE LAUDER PURE COLOUR LONG-LASTING LIPSTICK
Best lasting lipstick
£14 for 3.8g
Intense, high-shine colour that lasts, enhanced with vitamins C and E and the delicate fragrance of fresh fig. It won't leave a trace behind on your coffee cup!

GUERLAIN DIVINORA COLOUR AND SHINE LIPSTICK
Best for shine
£14 for 8ml
A glamorously packaged, creamy lipstick, enhanced with a golden shine to give lips a fuller appearance. Perfect for adding evening glamour.

LANCOME LIP DIMENSION
Best for true colours
£13.50 for 5.5g
Smooth and long-lasting, in elegant packaging, this lipstick uses volatile oils to ensure that the colour stays true and vibrant.

L'OREAL COLOUR RICHE
Best hydrating budget lipstick
£7.29 for 10g
A creamy product that lasts as long as designer lipsticks, but without the price tag. It is smudge-proof, fade-proof and kiss-proof and contains jojoba oil for a rich, silky finish.

MAX FACTOR LIPFINITY
Best long-lasting budget lipstick
£9.99 for 4.2ml
This product involves an innovative two-step process – apply the colour, then a moisturizing topcoat to seal it. It gives lips a glossy finish that lasts for up to eight hours, even when you eat and drink. It has to be taken off with eye make-up remover, yet doesn't leave lips dry.

MOLTON BROWN WONDER LIPS LIPLIFT FORMULA
Best long-term lip plumper
£23 for 1.5ml
Infused with vitamins C and E, this lipstick is designed to stimulate the lips' production of collagen after just 29 days. Gives a fuller appearance if used regularly.

NARS LIPSTICK
Best colour range
£15.50 for 3.4g
The creamy, easy-to-wear texture and vibrant high fashion colours make this a great buy. Intense moisturizers help soften the lips while adding rich colour. Choose from three formulas based on different finishes – sheer for a natural look, semi-matt for full-bodied, velvety lips and satin for creamy, shiny lips.

ORIGINS LASTING LIP COLOUR
Best scented lipstick
£10 for 3g
This creamy lipstick provides good definition that lasts. It is enriched with vitamin E and invigoratingly scented with mint.

REVLON COLOURSTAY LIP COLOUR
Best for longevity
£7.99 for 4g
The original extended-wear lipstick still stands tall among its peers. The uniquely patented formula contains vitamin E and aloe to condition. While it has a slightly dry texture, it lasts for hours. Available in 42 shades.

TIPS

- For lipstick that lasts all day, line lips with a pencil first, then colour in with the pencil and finally apply lipstick over the top.
- If you have thin lips, avoid matt textures as they can make your lips appear smaller. Choose a gloss colour instead and apply generously to the bottom lip.
- Never wear a darker lip pencil with a light lipstick.
- Using a lip primer before lip colour will prevent bleeding and provide a smooth, hydrated base for the colour to adhere to .

SHISEIDO STAYING POWER MOISTURIZING LIPSTICK
Best glossy lipstick
£15 for 3g
With ten times more glycerine than any other lipstick, colour stays glossy all day and lips are kept moisturized and soft.

SHISEIDO SHEER GLOSS LIPSTICK
Best sheer lipstick
£14 for 4g
A cross between a lipstick and a gloss, this sheer formula adds a hint of tint and shine to the lips. Try Honey Tea for a universally flattering, natural look.

YVES SAINT LAURENT ROUGE VIBRATION LIPSTICK
Best reds
£17 for 2g
This lipstick is available in 12 moisture-packed shades, sleekly packaged to ooze Parisian chic. The classic red is a must for evening sophistication.

LIP GLOSSES

AWAKE STARDOM LIP GLOSS
Best for hydrating
£12 for 7g
Deeply hydrating, this formula uses new 'Ice Flake' technology, whereby water is released when lips are pressed together, giving smoother, enviably fuller-looking lips. It also contains soothing extracts of watercress, jojoba oil and vitamin E.

BLOOM LIP GLOSS WAND
Best for conditioning
£9.95 for 8g
This conditions and moisturizes with essential oils while delivering an incredible high-shine gloss. Choose from eight subtle colours.

BOURJOIS EFFET 3D HIGH SHINE LIP COLOUR
Best budget lip gloss
£6.75 for 6.5ml
Available in 15 shades, this high-shine gloss can be used on naked lips, or over lipstick to create the illusion of fuller lips. This is top quality at an amazing price.

CHRISTIAN DIOR DIORIFIC PLASTIC SHINE
Best for an ultra-glossy finish
£13 for 5.5g
A reflective 'shine booster' is Dior's secret weapon for delivering a superglossy pout that lasts remarkably well. Choose from ten classic shades.

CLARINS CRYSTAL LIPGLOSS
Best clear gloss
£9 for 8ml
Elegantly packaged, this clear, smooth gloss gives an excellent sheen and stays moist for a long time. For grown-up lips with an intriguing gleam.

CLINIQUE GLOSSWEAR AND BRUSH (SPF 8)
Best natural-looking gloss
£9 for 5.8g
This cute pot of gloss comes with its own lip brush and adds a subtle, non-sticky sheen to lips. It comes in eight shades: try Air Kiss, a slightly iridescent pale pink, for a fresh, natural look.

DUWOP LIP VENOM
Best lip plumper
£14.50 for 3ml
For bee-stung lips that look naturally plump, this works by increasing circulation to the lip area and contains moisturizing jojoba and avocado oils. Wear over lip colour for extra shine.

ELIZABETH ARDEN EIGHT HOUR CREAM
Best all-round balm
£18 for 650ml
A fabulous all-purpose product, this makes an excellent lip gloss on top of colour, but can also be used to highlight the face. It is a classic that calms, restores, protects, heals and moisturizes cracked lips, skin irritations, cuticles and even dry elbows.

LANCOME JUICY TUBES
Best sheer colours
£11.50 for 6ml
These fruit-flavoured ultra-shine glosses taste as good as they look and give a brilliant transparent, lacquered effect. The palette is updated seasonally and the range is always a sellout.

L'OREAL GLAM SHINE
Best sparkly lip gloss
£6.99 for 10g
This ultra-shimmery liquid lipstick plumps up the lips and instantly transforms your look for evening with eyecatching sparkle.

MAC LIPGLASS
Best high-shine gloss
£9.50 for 9ml
Only a tiny amount of this thickly textured gloss is needed to give your lips a luminous look and great shine. It's a favourite of make-up artists.

POUT LIP POLISH
Best for luscious gloss
£10 for 7.5ml
This chic compact is filled with supershiny dense gloss for lusciously kissable lips.
Available in eight shades.

SISLEY BOTANICAL LIPGLOSS
Best for protecting
£16 for 10ml
A transparent, shiny gloss that gives a fabulous gleam, and contains calendula
extracts and shea butter to moisturize and protect lips.

STILA LIP GLAZE
Best for celebrity gloss
£18 for 5ml
This ultra-shiny, fruit-flavoured gloss in a twist-up pen – and with a brush – comes
from a brand founded by make-up artist Jeanine Lobel and beloved of celebrities.

ULTIMA II EXTRAORDINAIRE VOLUMIZING LIP GLOSS (SPF 6)
Best volumizing gloss
£13.50 for 5ml
Nourishing ingredients include vitamin E and wheatgerm and sesame oils, while
light-reflecting properties ensure a seriously glossy shine.

URBAN DECAY SHINE GLOSS
Best funky colours
£10.50 for 12ml
This is superglossy and feels fabulous on the lips. It comes in an irresistible range
of funky, glittery colours. Brilliant for creating dramatic impact.

NAIL POLISHES

BOURJOIS SHOCK RESISTANT NAIL ENAMEL
Best hardwearing polish
£4.95 for 12ml
Enriched with calcium and pro-vitamin B5 to make it chip-proof for days, this
glossy polish contains a hint of pearl and is available in all the latest colours.

CHANEL NAIL LACQUER
Best for a 'straight-off-the-catwalk' look
£11.50 for 13ml
Durable and dazzlingly shiny, Chanel's legendary nail colours are updated
seasonally with the catwalk trends. Try the classic Flamme Rose for a natural
sheen, or the bestselling Rouge Noir for a dramatic look.

CHRISTIAN DIOR DIOR ADDICT ONE-COAT NAIL COLOR
Best natural shades
£11.50 for 14.5ml
Available in a huge range of colours, from the most subtle to the most flamboyant, Dior's long-lasting polishes really do only need one coat. They also have a great, glossy finish.

CREATIVE NAIL DESIGN IN 'STICKY'
Best for making polish last longer
£8.95 for 14ml
Apply this undercoat before your polish for long-lasting results – the base acts as adhesive so that polish sticks and doesn't peel or chip off.

CREATIVE NAIL DESIGN IN 'SUPER SHINY'
Best topcoat for a shiny finish
£8.95 for 14ml
This high-gloss, super-hard topcoat dries quickly and protects your nail polish, helping it to last up to three weeks.

ESSIE IN 'ALLURE'
Best everyday polish
£7.99 for 12ml
This is a natural shade, not too white or too pink. It works with any skin tone to give nails a transparent, healthy glow with extra sparkle.

ESTEE LAUDER PURE COLOUR NAIL LACQUER
Best luxury polish
£11 for 9ml
A high-tech formula that gives a long-lasting shine to your nails. It comes in a rich choice of colours and the ice-cube-style glass bottles will look gorgeous on your dressing table.

GUERLAIN COLOUR AND SHINE NAIL ENAMEL
Best for high-gloss finish
£12 for 9.5ml
Made with an impact-resistant formula to impart even coverage and conceal ridges and imperfections, the polish has a particularly smooth texture that makes it is easy to apply. Choose from 22 shiny shades.

HARD CANDY NAIL POLISH
Best funky colours
£9.95 for 12ml
Thankfully, these ever-popular nail polishes now come in a new, longer-lasting formulation. Choose from 25 fantastic glittery, matt and sheer colours, each with a funky plastic ring.

L'OREAL PERFECTION JET SET NAIL
Best fast-drying nail varnish
£4.99 for 12ml

When you have little time on your hands a fast-drying nail polish is vital. Jet Set Nail dries in just 60 seconds – simply apply one coat, wait one minute and you are ready to go with no need for a second coat. The fast-drying formula also enables an even distribution of colour particles to give brilliant colour and a high-gloss finish.

MAC CREAM NAIL POLISH
Best for bright colours
£7 for 14ml

This high-shine polish wears well and also offers a huge variety of fashionable colours. Depending on the look you are after, you can choose from classic matt or high shine.

OPI NAIL LACQUER
Best for a professional finish
£8 for 14ml

Available in a wide variety of vibrant and intense shades, these lacquers, with silk proteins, are favoured by many manicurists and celebrities as they last incredibly well and don't chip easily.

REVLON NAIL ENAMEL
Best for variety
£6.29 for 15ml

Spectacularly glossy, this protective polish contains a fortifying complex and comes in a range of classic shades. It goes on smoothly and is very hard wearing. Available in 33 chip-resistant shades.

YVES SAINT LAURENT PURE NAIL LACQUER
Best for glamour
£13.50 for 9ml

A rich formula that is available in a brilliant range of sophisticated shades. The deep reds are perfect for creating Parisian-chic nails.

MAKE-UP PALETTES

BENEFIT GLAMOURETTE
Best three-in-one product
£32.50

This 1940s-style make-up set oozes retro chic for that vintage look and consists of a double compact with blusher on one side and face powder on the other, plus a coordinating lipstick in the handle.

CHANEL ESSENTIE DE CHANEL
Best for timeless glamour
£28
A timeless classic, this wonderfully elegant compact contains six classic shades for eyes, cheeks and lips. The iridescent gold is marvellous for adding gloss to lips and lids alike. It comes with two good-quality brush applicators to ensure precise application.

EYEKO MAKE-OUT
Best for travel
£15
This pocket-sized pink palette from the cult Japanese brand cleverly swivels open to reveal two eyeshadows, a blusher, lip gloss and a double-ended sponge applicator. This is a great space-saving product for the handbag or perfect for taking on weekends away.

NARS MAKE-UP COMPACT
Best for versatility
£52
Four eyeshadows, two blushers and four lip colours are contained in this sleek, black, stylish palette. It comes in many evocatively-named colour combinations, and you can choose from a range in natural shades to a selection of funkier, brighter colours.

TRISH MCEVOY MAXED OUT LIP GLOSS KIT
Best handbag-size lip kit
£18
Amazingly compact, this kit contains everything you might need to fix your lips when you are out. Ten universally flattering shades of Trish McEvoy's famous lip colours and glosses are packed into this tiny, credit card-sized compact. It comes complete with a mirror and mini lip brush for easy application.

SMASHBOX SMOKEBOX
Best eyeshadow palette
£30
This is the only eye palette you'll ever need: a collection of ten easy-to-blend eyeshadows, comprised of five matt shades on one side with matching shimmer shades on the opposite side.

URBAN DECAY FACE CASE
Best for parties
£20
The perfect accessory for girls on the go, this multifunctional compact comes with eight funky, glittery eye, lip and cheek colours, plus a double-ended applicator and mirror.

MAKE-UP BRUSHES

BECCA FOUNDATION BRUSH NO.18
Best synthetic foundation brush
£28
This brush is made from an exclusive nonabsorbent fibre, so that your liquid, cream or stick foundation applies perfectly evenly.

BECCA POWDER AND BRONZER BRUSH
Best for blending powder
£35 (medium, no.15) or £40 (large, no.16)
Made from racoon fibres, this superfine handmade brush is great for picking up loose powder and dispersing it easily.

BECCA SMALL CONCEALER BRUSH NO.3
Best concealer brush
£18
Made from a synthetic fibre called toray, this brush has a fine, pointed tip to give accuracy and control when covering flaws and blemishes.

BENEFIT GEL BENT EYE LINER BRUSH
Best eyeliner brush
£11
The natural fibres and fine texture make this the essential tool for applying liquid eyeliner smoothly and accurately.

BOBBI BROWN BROW BRUSH
Best natural brow brush
£32
The angled head of this brush expertly shapes and defines natural-looking brows. Made from bevelled goat and pony hair, this delicate brush is ideal for adding the finishing touches to your brows.

THE BODY SHOP BRUSHES
Best budget brushes
£5 – £12
This good-quality and yet affordable range has every brush you might need, from a lipstick/concealer brush to a face/body brush. Made from supersoft synthetic fibres, they have a tapered shape.

GIORGIO ARMANI BROW AND LASH BRUSH
Best synthetic brow brush
£12
Made from synthetic bristles, this is the ideal tool for both neatening your eyebrows and combing through mascara, for a well-groomed look.

▦ MAC 150 LARGE POWDER BRUSH
Best for applying loose powder
£30
A large, domed brush made from goat fibres, this has a particularly soft texture that holds and disperses powder extremely well and so is brilliant for applying face powder evenly.

▦ MISTER MASCARA FOLDING LASH COMB
Best lash and eyebrow comb
£5
Use this to comb lashes through after you have applied your mascara. It effectively removes any clumps of extra mascara and pulls lashes into perfect shape. It is also handy for taming unruly eyebrows.

▦ MISTER MASCARA MULTI BRUSH
Best multipurpose brush
£12.50
This goat-hair blusher brush contains three mini brushes in the handle: a lip brush, an eyeliner brush and an eyeshadow brush, made from both sable and synthetic fibres. This ingenious tool is small enough to fit in your handbag and can be used to apply all your make-up.

▦ PRESCRIPTIVES FOUNDATION BRUSH
Best natural foundation brush
£32
A luxurious brush that is made from the finest quality sable, and will blend your foundation flawlessly.

▦ SCREENFACE MINI APPLICATOR
Best mascara wand
£4.95
This magic wand is unbeatable for combing through lashes after applying mascara to prevent clumping.

▦ SHU UEMURA 6M SABLE LIP BRUSH
Best natural lip brush
£15.50
Its long, slim handle and oval-shaped tip means that this high-quality brush gives impressive definition and fills in lipstick flawlessly.

▦ SHU UEMURA 18R POWDER BRUSH
Best natural powder brush
£32
This full brush has a medium texture as it is made with pony hair, enabling you to blend bronzer or powder effortlessly into the face.

TONY AND TINA POWDER BRUSH
Best synthetic powder brush
£70
If you prefer not to use products made from animal hair, this soft, synthetic brush with a long, clear handle and rounded tip is the one.

URBAN DECAY LIP BRUSH
Best synthetic lip brush
£13
The synthetic bristles and small handle make for expert lipstick application.

YVES SAINT LAURENT NO.3 SHADOW BLENDER
Best eyeshadow brush
£16
Marten bristles form an oval shape for blending eyeshadow seamlessly. It is especially good for smudging colour along the crease of the eye.

TOOLS

BLINC CURL HEATED EYELASH CURLER
Best for long-lasting curly lashes
£14.50
A simple-to-use heated eyelash curler that shapes lashes in seconds, giving them wonderfully long-lasting curves. It works without clamping and requires only the tiniest amount of pressure.

CHANEL SHARPENER
Best sharpener for eye and lip pencils
£ N/A
Unfortunately these sharpeners are not sold separately from Chanel's eye pencils (£13) and lip pencils (£14.50). They are, however, by far the best sharpeners on the market so well-worth investing in.

DIAMANCEL FOOT FILE
Best for smoothing feet
£29 to £39
A hardcore home-pedicure accessory, this industrial-strength foot file removes hardened skin from the heels fast. Apply foot cream straight after for silky feet.

MAC BRUSH CLEANER
Best brush cleaner
£6 for 235ml
Ensure your brushes last longer by cleaning them regularly with this potion that cleanses, disinfects and conditions the fibres.

MEDIC CUCUMBER CLEAN-UP STICK
Best for correcting eye make-up
£14.95
This handy pencil cleans away mascara or eyeliner mistakes in seconds, without you having to rub at the delicate eye area and make it red. It also contains cucumber to soothe and refresh skin.

MISTER MASCARA JAPANESE POINT TWEEZERS
Best for perfectionists
£16.99
A stainless steel tweezer that is excellent for removing difficult and hard-to-see hairs. One for the perfectionists.

OPTREX EYE DEW BLUE EYE DROPS
Best cosmetic eye drops
£3.95 for 10ml
For tired, bloodshot, red or dry eyes, this is a quick fix. Keep for special occasions or emergencies; it's not meant to be used for more than three consecutive days.

RUBY & MILLIE PERFECT NAIL PEN
Best for correcting nail polish
£4.50
An ingenious pen that has a small felt-tip loaded with nail polish remover, so that you can remove unwanted nail-polish smears or smudges with accuracy.

SHU UEMURA LASH CURLER
Best for curling eyelashes
£16
This bestseller is found in many make-up artists' tool bags, as it is so light and easy to use. The rubber inside the curler is rounded so that it curls lashes perfectly to give an eye-opening effect that lasts all day, with or without mascara.

TWEEZERMAN SLANT TWEEZERS
Best for tweezing eyebrows
£16
These classic tweezers are essential for creating perfectly arched brows, and come with a lifetime guarantee so that when they go blunt you can send them back to be sharpened.

TWEEZERMAN CUTICLE NIPPERS
Best for keeping cuticles in check
£14.50
Chrome-plated and made from hardened steel, the blade is matt and cuts at the very tip, while the double spring ensures that they operate smoothly. They should last for ever.

UK TOP TEN BEST HIGH STREET BUYS

If the idea of braving the beauty counters at a large department store is an altogether too exhausting a task to contemplate for a Saturday morning, or you're still trying to pay off your credit card from holiday extravagances, then why not hit the high street? Many pharmacies and supermarkets have some great-quality beauty products that offer excellent quality and value for money. Although these own-label brands vary from country to country, here is a list of some of the best products that are available in the UK for under £15.

BOOTS BOTANICS RADIANCE BOOSTER
Best skin highlighter
£9 for 40ml
If you are a fan of Clarin's Beauty Flash Balm, then you will love this product. Enriched with skin-protecting apple and pure extract of wheatgerm, to condition and help maintain the elasticity of the skin, it revitalizes and moisturizes tired skin for instant rejuvenation. The addition of light-diffusing pearls also gives the complexion an illuminated glow.

BOOTS NO. 7 INTELLIGENT COLOUR FOUNDATION
Best foundation for all skin tones
£3 per 10ml
An ultra-lightweight formula that won't block pores, this foundation glides easily onto the skin and contains vitamins A and E to protect and condition. Choose from three shades – light, medium and dark – after application, the colour miraculously adapts to the skin's natural tone.

CAPSULE PICK ME UP MASK
Best mask for all skin types, especially sensitive
£14 for 75ml
A superhydrating mask with a zingy citrus aroma to boost even the most stressed-out skin. Packed full of powerful restoratives, moisturizing algae extract, mint water and chamomile, it soothes and revives the face without irritation. The mask goes on smoothly and is easy to rinse off.

MARKS AND SPENCER AUTOGRAPH SOFT POWDER BLUSH
Best blush
£11 for 6g
This superfine powder blush delivers colour evenly to the cheeks and is also easy to layer to create a subtle or stronger effect. It is also hypoallergenic, comes packaged in a sleek, mirrored compact and is available in ten great shades from sunglow to cinnabar.

MARKS AND SPENCER ORGANIC EXTRACTS PROTECTIVE DAY MOISTURIZER
Best day cream
£8 for 50ml
Composed of 95 per cent organic ingredients, this light day cream contains a blend of soothing aloe vera, as well as a natural antioxidant complex of green tea and lycopene, which helps to moisten and protect.

MEA EYESHADOW
Best eyeshadow range
from £6
As part of a cosmetic collection that is exclusive to Debenhams, MEA eyeshadow has a soft, velvety texture that blends gently into the lids. Shadows are available in a huge variety of colours, such as twilight, frosty blue and lilac shimmer, and you can choose from matt, frost or glitter finishes.

RIMMEL LASTING FINISH LIPSTICK
Best non-smudge lipstick
£3.49 for 5ml
High-lustre and long lasting, this lipstick formula contains a blend of skin conditioners. Polybutene improves shine and the adhesion of colour pigments to the lips, and panthenol (pro-vitamin B), vitamin E and candelilla wax act as a barrier to retain water. The lipstick glides on easily and won't smudge. It is available in more than 20 colours.

SAINSBURY'S ACTIVE NATURALS BALANCING SHAMPOO
Best shampoo
£1.99 for 250ml
This natural-ingredient shampoo contains antioxidant green tea and celery extract to detoxify and cleanse. It gives life to dull, lacklustre locks.

TESCO MAKE-UP CONCEALER
Best concealer
£4.99 for 1.6g
Make-up artist Barabara Daly has created a cosmetics range exclusive to Tesco supermarkets. This creamy concealer blends in easily and, being based on yellow tones, works well with most skin tones, from fair to dark. It provides longlasting coverage that camouflages blemishes, dark circles and broken capillaries.

TESCO SKIN WISDOM BODY LOTION
Best body moisturizer
£1.99 for 300ml
By Bharti Vyas for Tesco, this body moisturizer is enriched with soothing chamomile, green tea, shea butter, manoi oil and allantoin. A deeply invigorating lotion, it smoothes effortlessly into the skin, leaving it soft.

THE DIRECTORY

Use this list of websites, telephone numbers and addresses to help you track down your chosen product or to seek further advice or information from specialist organizations. Major brand contacts are also included to help you to find local stockists, store locations and mail order.

UK

DEPARTMENT STORES, BOUTIQUES AND PHARMACIES

BOOTS GROUP PLC
1 Thane Road
Nottingham NG2 3AA
Tel: 0845 0708090
www.boots-plc.com
www.wellbeing.com

BOUTIQUE CARTIER
188 Sloane Street
London SW1X 9QR
Tel: 020 7235 9023
Tel: 020 7408 5700 for stockists

COSMETICS A LA CARTE LTD
18 Motcomb Street
London SW1X 8LB
Tel: 020 7622 2318 for mail order
www.cosmeticsalacarte.com

CRABTREE AND EVELYN
27 Kelso Place
London W8 5QG
Tel: 020 7361 0499

THE CROWN PERFUMERY COMPANY
51 Burlington Arcade
London SW1Y 4EL
Tel: 020 7839 3434

DEBENHAMS
Stores nationwide, including:
334-348 Oxford Street
London W1C 1JG
Tel: 020 7580 3000
0845 6055044 customer helpline
www.debenhams.com

DICKINS AND JONES
224 Regent Street
London W1A 1DB
Tel: 020 7734 7070

ETRO
14 Old Bond Street
London W1X 3DB
Tel: 020 7495 5767

FENWICK
63 New Bond Street
London W1A 3BS
Tel: 020 7629 9161
www.fenwick.co.uk

FORTNUM & MASON
181 Piccadilly
London W1A 1ER
Tel: 020 7734 8040
www.fortnumandmason.com

HARRODS HAIR AND BEAUTY
Knightsbridge
London SW1X 7XL
Tel: 020 7730 1234
www.harrods.com

HARVEY NICHOLS
109–25 Knightsbridge
London SW1X 7RJ
Tel: 020 7235 5000
www.harveynichols.com

HERMES LONDON
155 New Bond Street
London W1Y 9PA
Tel: 020 7499 8856

HOUSE OF FRASER
Head Office: 1 Howick Place
London SW1P 1BH
Tel: 020 7963 2000
www.houseoffraser.co.uk

JO MALONE
150 Sloane Street
London SW1X 9BX
Tel: 020 7730 2100

JOHN LEWIS
22 stores nationwide including:
278-306 Oxford Street
London W1A 1EX
Tel: 020 7629 7711

KIEHL'S
29 Monmouth Street
London WC2 9DD
Tel: 020 7240 2411 for enquiries
and mail order

L'ARTISAN PARFUMEUR
17 Cale Street
London SW3 3OR
Tel: 020 7352 4196

LES SENTEURS
227 Ebury Street
London SW1W 8UT
Tel: 020 7730 2322

LIBERTY
210–220 Regent Street
London W1R 6AH
Tel: 020 7734 1234
www.liberty.co.uk

L'OCCITANE LIMITED
15-19 Cavendish Place
London W1G 0QE
Tel: 020 7907 0300
www.loccitane.com

MAC COSMETICS
28 Fouberts Place
West Soho
London W1F 7PR
Tel: 020 7534 9222
www.maccosmetics.com

MAKE UP FOR EVER
51 South Molton Street
London W1K 5SD
Tel: 020 7529 5690
www.makeupforever.com

MASON PEARSON BROS LTD
37 Old Bond Street
London W1X 4HL
Tel: 020 7491 2613

MOLTON BROWN COSMETICS
58 South Molton Street
London W1K 5SL
Tel: 020 7499 6474
www.moltonbrown.com

NEAL'S YARD NATURAL REMEDIES
15 Neal's Yard
London WC2H 9DP
Tel: 020 7379 7222
www.nealsyardremedies.com

PENHALIGON'S
Flagship store: 41 Wellington Street
London WC2E 7BN
Tel: 020 7836 2150
Tel: 0800 716108 for stores nationwide
and mail order
www.penhaligons.co.uk

PIXI
22a Fouberts Place
London W1F 7PW
Tel: 020 7287 7211

PLANET ORGANIC
42 Westbourne Grove
London W2 5SH
Tel: 020 7221 7171
www.planetorganic.com

POUT
32 Shelton Street
London WC2H 9JE
Tel: 020 7379 0379
www.pout.co.uk

RALPH LAUREN
Flagship store: 1 New Bond Street
London W1S 3RL
Tel: 020 7535 4600
Tel: 0141 242 6000

REN
Head office tel: 020 7724 2900
40 Liverpool Street
London EC2M 7QN
Tel: 020 7618 5353

SCREEN FACE
48 Monmouth Street
London WC2 9EP
Tel: 020 7836 3955
www.screenface.com

SELFRIDGES
400 Oxford Street
London W1A 1AB
Tel: 020 7629 1234
www.selfridges.com

SEPHORA
63 Gee Street
London EC1V 3RS
Tel: 020 7253 2194
www.sephora.com

SHU UEMURA
Unit 15–16 Thomas Neal's
41 Earlham Street
London WC2 9LD
Tel: 020 7379 6627

SPACE NK
Head office: 200 Great Portland Street
London W1W 5QG
Tel: 020 7299 4999 for branches
nationwide
Tel: 0870 169 9999 for mail order
www.spacenk.co.uk

HOME SHOPPING WEBSITES

www.auravita.com
www.beautycenter.co.uk
www.buycosmeticsdirect.com/ub4
www.cosmeticbargains.co.uk
www.creativenailplace.com
www.dealtime.co.uk
www.escentual.co.uk
www.eskaye.co.uk
www.estoreuk.com/beauty-product/index.html
www.fascination-perfumery.co.uk
www.fragrancebay.com
www.garden.co.uk
www.health-store.co.uk
www.highcheekbones.com
www.interscent.co.uk
www.lookfantastic.com
www.missgroovy.co.uk
www.perfuma.com
www.pharmacy2u.co.uk
www.saveonmakeup.co.uk
www.spacenk.co.uk
www.stores.ebay.co.uk
www.wellbeing.com

REGULATING BODIES, PROFESSIONAL SOCIETIES AND ASSOCIATIONS

THE BRITISH ASSOCIATION OF DERMATOLOGISTS
19 Fitzroy Square
London W1P 5HQ
Tel: 020 7383 0266
www.bad.org.uk

THE COSMETIC TOILETRY AND PERFUMERY ASSOCIATION (CTPA) LIMITED
Josaron House
5/7 John Princes Street
London W1G 0JN
Tel: 020 7491 8891
www.ctpa.org.uk

PHILIP KINGSLEY TRICHOLOGY
54 Green Street
London W1K 6RU
Tel: 020 7629 4004
www.philipkingsley.co.uk

THE TRICHOLOGICAL SOCIETY
19 Balgores Square
Gidea Park, near. Romford
Essex RM2 6AU
United Kingdom
Tel: 01708 728980
www.hairscientists.org

PRODUCT REVIEW/TESTING AND INFORMATION WEBSITES

www.allergyfoundation.com
www.beautyconsumer.com
www.ciao.co.uk
www.cosmetiquenews.com
www.ctpa.org.uk (Cosmetic Toiletry & Perfumery Association)
www.dermatology.co.uk

www.dooyoo.co.uk/lifestyle
www.dti.gov.uk/access/cosmetic
(Department of Trade and Industry – Cosmetic Product Regulations)
www.hair2stay.co.uk
www.handbag.com/beauty
www.ifscc.org (International Federation of Societies of Cosmetic Chemists)
www.iso.ch (International Organization for Standardization (ISO))
www.marshmallow.co.uk/reviews/
www.reviewcentre.com
www.tradingstandards.gov.uk
www.trial.which.co.uk
www.trichology.co.uk
www.trichology.uk.com

USA

DEPARTMENT STORES, BOUTIQUES AND PHARMACIES

ALEXANDER PERFUMES AND COSMETICS
7914 Girard Avenue
La Jolla, CA 92037
Tel: 858 454 2292 or 800 326 1632
www.beautyandscents.com

ANNA SUI
275 West 39th Street, Fifth Floor
New York NY 10018
Tel: 212 768 1004
Tel: 212 941 8406 for stockists

APOTHIA
Brentwood Gardens
11677 San Vicente Blvd
Brentwood, CA 90049
Tel: 310 207 8411
www.apothia.com

AVEDA SALON & SPA
456 West Broadway
New York NY 10012
Tel: 212 473 0280
Tel: 866 823 1425 for nearest store
www.aveda.com

BABETTE
924 1/2 Massachusetts Street
Lawrence, KS 66044
Tel: 866 749 2227
www.babette.net

BARNEYS
Stores nationwide including:
New York
660 Madison Avenue
New York, NY 10021
Tel: 212 826 8900

also at: Beverly Hills
9570 Wilshire Boulevard
Beverly Hills, CA
Tel: 310 276 4400

Also 12 outlet stores including:
1420 Fifth Avenue
Seattle, WA
Tel: 206 622 6300
www.barneys.com

BARTELL DRUGS
Flagship store: 600 1st Ave N
Seattle WA 98109-4001
Tel: 206 284 1353
Tel: 877 227 8355 for information
www.bartelldrugs.com

A BEAUTIFUL LIFE
9 West Bridge Street
New Hope, PA 18938
Tel: 866 862

BERGDORF GOODMAN
754 Fifth Ave
New York, NY 10019
Tel: 212 872 2750
Tel: 800 558 1855 for enquiries

BEYOND THE PALE
22 E. Washington Street
Middleburg
VA 20118
Tel: 540 687 8050

BLISS SPA
569 Broadway
New York NY 10012
Tel: 212 219 8970
www.blissworld.com

BLOOMINGDALE'S
Tel: 800 777 4999
Stores nationwide including:
59th Street and Lexington Ave
1000 3rd Avenue
New York, NY 10022
Tel: 212 705 2000
www.bloomingdales.com

WILLOW GROVE PARK MALL
2400 Moreland Park
Willow Grove PA 19090
Tel: 215 706 3300

1 STANFORD SHOPPING CENTER
Palo Alto CA 94304
Tel: 650 463 2000

THE FALLS MALL
8778 SW 136th Street
Miami FL 33176
Tel: 305 252 6300

600 N. WABASH
Chicago IL 60611
Tel: 312 324 7500

CENTURY CITY SHOPPING CENTER
10250 Santa Monica Boulevard
Los Angeles CA 90067
Tel: 310 772 2100

THE FASHION SHOW
3200 Las Vegas Avenue
Las Vegas NV 89109
Tel: 702 784 5400
www.bloomingdales.com

BLUEMERCURY
Retail store in Philadelphia, New Jersey and Washington DC including:
Georgetown
3059 M Street NW
Washington, DC 20007
Tel: 202 965 1300
Tel: 800 355 6000
www.bluemercury.com

BOBBI BROWN ESSENTIALS
600 Madison Ave
New York
NY 10022
Tel: 212 980 7040
www.bobbibrowncosmetics.com

THE BODY SHOP INC (USA)
5036 One World Way Wake Forest
North Carolina 27587 USA
Tel: 919 554 4900
www.thebodyshop.com

THE BON MARCHE
Stores in five states including:
918 W. Idaho Street
Boise, ID 83702-5715
Tel: 208 388 7000

15340 N.E. 24th Street
Redmond, WA 98052-5528
Tel: 425 688 6850

501 Wyoming Blvd
Casper, WY 82609-4220
Tel: 307 268 6000
Tel: 866 464 8787 for internet
customer service
www.thebon.com

**BOUTIQUE GIORGIO ARMANI
NEW YORK**
760 Madison Avenue
New York, NY 10021
Tel: 212 988 9191

BROWNES & CO APOTHECARY
841 Lincoln Road
Miami Beach, FL 33139
Tel: 888 BROWNES
www.brownesbeauty.com

BURDINES
Stores statewide including:
7801 Citrus Park Town Center
Tampa, FL 33625-3178
Tel: 813 926 7300
Tel: 800 334 7467 for home shopping
and customer care

3800 US Hwy 98 North
Suite 400
Lakeland, FL 33809-3833
Tel: 941 853 7200
www.burdines.com

C O BIGELOW
414 Sixth Ave
near 9th Street
New York, NY 10011
Tel: 212 533 2700
Tel: 800 793 5433 for mail order

COLORS-N-SCENTS
21 N. Main Street
Butte
MT 59701
Tel: 888 785 0926
www.colour-sens.com

COS BAR
309 South Galena
Aspen, CO 81611
Tel: 970 925 6249
Tel: 800 722 8982 to order
www.thecosbar.com

COSMETIQUE BEAUTY CENTER
Woodbury Commons Shopping Center
8285 Jericho Turnpike
Woodbury, NY 11797
Tel: 800 892 5320
www.cosmetiquebeauty.com

CVS PHARMACY
Flagship Store: 256 237 7683
Stores nationwide including:
1629 Quintard Ave
Anniston, AL 36201
Tel: 888 607 4287 for customer care
www.cvs.com

**DOCTOR'S DERMALOGIC
FORMULA DDF, INC.**
99 Calvert Street
Harrison, NY 10528
Tel: 914 835 2200

DUANE READE INC.
East coast chemists with stores including:
440 Ninth Ave, 6th Floor
New York, NY 10001
Tel: 212 273 5700
www.duanereade.com

E6 APOTHECARY
167 Newbury Street
Boston
MA 02116
Tel: 617 236 8138 (local)
Tel: 1 800 664 6635 (toll free)
www.e6apothecary.com

ENVIE
328 Heymann Blvd Lafayette
LA 70503
Tel: 337 261 9737

EYEKO STOCKED BY:
Maximum Cosmetics & Eyebeauty.com
506 1/2 N. Sweetzer Ave
Los Angeles, CA 90048
Tel: 1 800 89 EYEKO
www.eyebeautyusa.com

FILLMORE BOUTIQUE
2117 Fillmore Street
(@ California Street)
San Francisco, CA 94115
Tel: 415 567 0242

FRANCIS JEROME
124 South 19th Street
Philadelphia, PA 19103
Tel: 215 988 0440
www.FJBeauty.com

FRED SEGAL
8100 Melrose Ave. at Crescent Heights
West Hollywood, California 90046
Tel: 323 651 4129
www.fredsegalbeauty.com

GEMAYEL
2030 Broadway (at 70th Street)
New York, NY 10023
Tel: 212 787 5555
www.gemayelspa.com

GLENPRO BEAUTY CENTER, INC
717 E. California Ave
Glendale CA 91206
Tel: 818-244-8776
www.glenprobeauty.com

GLO
180 Steele Street
Denver
CO 80206
Tollfree 1 800 462 5790
www.gloskincare.com

GOLDSMITH'S
Six locations in Tennesee, including:
Highway 45 South
Jackson, TN 38305-4915
Tel: 901 668 6393
www.goldsmiths.com

HENRI BENDEL
712 5th Ave New York
NY 10019-4108
Tel: 212 247 1100
Tel: 800 423 6335 for customer care
www.henribendel.com

JO MALONE
949 Broadway
New York, NY 10010
Tel: 212 673 2220

KANEBO COSMETICS USA, INC.
693 Fifth Avenue, 17th Floor
New York, NY 10022
Tel: 866 271 6815 for orders

KIEHL'S
109 Third Ave
near 13th St
New York, NY
Tel: 212 677 3171
Tel: 1 800 543 4572 for customer services

LAZARUS
Head office tel: 770 913 4000
77 stores in nine states, including:
3919 Lafayette Road
Indianapolis, IN 46254-2531
Tel: 317 298 2205
7900 Shelbyville Rd.
Louisville, KY 40222-5451
Tel: 502 423 3200

400 Monroeville Mall
Monroeville, PA 15146
Tel: 412 858 3710

Unit #300 Huntington Mall
Barboursville, WV 25504-0001
Tel: 304 733 0205
www.lazarusonline.com

**LILY'S APOTHECARY
INSIDE THE HISTORIC
PLYMOUTH POST OFFICE
BUILDING**
6 Main Street Extension
Plymouth, MA 02360
Tel: 508 747 7546
www.lilysapothecary.com

LORD AND TAYLOR
85 stores nationwide including:
424 Fifth Ave
New York, NY
Tel: 212 391 3344
Tel: 1 800 223 7440 for telephone
orders

8001 South Orange Blossom Trail
Orlando, FL 32809
Tel: 407 851 6255

6000 Willowbrook Mall
Houston, TX 77070
Tel: 281 970 7900

LOUIS BOSTON
234 Berkeley Street
Boston, MA 02111
Tel: 800 225 5135
www.louisboston.com

MACY'S
Over 200 stores nationwide, including:
Macy's East
151 West 34th Street
New York, NY 10001 2101
Tel: 212 695 4400

Also at: Macy's West
1732 E. Shaw Avenue
Fresno, CA 93710-8104
Tel: 209 228 3333

Macy's East
6400 T. Springfield Mall
Springfield, VA 22150-1707
Tel: 703 719 6100

Macy's West
2727 Sage Road
Houston, TX 77056-5504
Tel: 800 289 6229 for phone orders
www.macys.com

MAKE UP FOR EVER
209 West Broadway
New York, NY 10012
Tel: 212 941 9337

MARSHALL FIELD'S
Tel: 1 800 634 3537 to order from
on-line advertisements
64 stores in the Upper Midwest
including:
111 N. State Street
Chicago, Illinois
Tel: 312 781 1000

700 Briarwood Cir
Ann Arbor, MI 48108-1614
Tel: 734 998 5000

600 Kirkwood Mall
Bismarck, ND 58504 5727
Tel: 701 255 5300

702 North Midvale Blvd
Madison, WI 53705
Tel: 608 232 2400
www.marshallfields.com

NAIMIE'S BEAUTY CENTER
12640 Riverside Dr.
Valley Village, CA 91607
Tel: 818 655 9933
www.naimies.com

NEIMAN MARCUS
Over 30 stores nationwide, including:
9700 Wilshire Boulevard
Beverly Hills, CA 90212
Tel: 310 550 5900 and 877 634 6263

3393 Peachtree Road NE
Atlanta, GA 30326
Tel: 404 266 8200 and 800 555 5077

1450 Ala Moana Boulevard
Honolulu , HI 96814
Tel: 808 951 8887 and 877 951 8887

5 Copley Place
Boston , MA 02116
Tel: 617 536 3660 and 877 563 4626

1200 Morris Turnpike
Short Hills, NJ 07078
Tel: 973 912 0080 and 877 777 5321
Tell: 800 937 9146
www.neimanmarcus.com

NORDSTROM
STORES NATIONWIDE
INCLUDING:
Westside Pavilion (#343)
10830 West Pico Boulevard
Los Angeles, CA 90064-2106
Tel: 310 470 6155

Dallas Galleria (#720)
5220 Alpha Road
Dallas, TX 75240-4316
Tel: 972 702 0055

Also at: The Westchester-White
Plains (#523)
135 Westchester Avenue
White Plains, NY 10601-4511
Tel: 914 946 1122
Tel: 888 282 6060 for customer service
www.nordstrom.com

OLE HENRIKSEN
8622 A West Sunset Boulevard
Los Angeles, California 90069-2301
Tel: 310 854 7700
www.olefacebody.com

PARFUMERIE DOUGLAS
Stores nationwide including:
Liberty Place, 1625 Chestnut St
Philadelphia, PA
Tel: 215 569 0770

Also at: 50 Massachusetts Avenue
Northeast
Washington, DC 20002
Tel: 202 789 1360

PARISIAN
Stores in Alabama, Florida, Georgia,
Indiania, Michigan, Mississippi, Ohio,
South Carolina and Tennesee, including:
1901 6th Ave N Suite 150
Birmingham, AL 35203
Tel: 205 581 0411

One West Washington Street
Indianapolis, IN 46204
Tel: 317 971 6200

1800 Galleria Blvd, St 5000
Franklin, TN 37067
Tel: 615 771 3200
www.parisian.com

PENHALIGON'S
870 Madison Avenue
New York, NY 10021
Tel: 212 249 1771

For mail order:
257 Union Street
Northvale, NJ 07647
Tel: 877 736 4254 or 201 767 7515
www.penhaligons.co.uk

PERFUMANIA
Stores nationwide including:
40A Serramonte Center Road
Daly City, CA 94015
Tel: 650 994 7145

Also at: 4800 Briarcliff Road NE,
Space#1024
Atlanta, GA 30345
Tel: 770 723 1404

560 West Prien Lake Road, Space #F8
St. Charles, LA 70601
Tel 337 562 8400

700 Haywood Road, PO Box 221, Unit
1033-A
Greenville, SC 29607
Tel: 864 676 9911

2882 D Third Ave
Bronx, NY 10455
Tel: 718 292 5893
www.perfumania.com

PRESCRIPTIVES
767 Fifth Ave
New York, NY 10153
Tel: 212 572 4400

PRETTY PRETTY COSMETICS
27 Park Place, Suite 200
New York, NY 10007
Tel: 866 773 8892
www.pretty2.com

PRIVAT PERFUMERY
980 N Michigan Ave # 1700
Chicago, IL 60611
Tel: 312 951 7000

PRIVATE EDITION
Graces Plaza
4009 Hillsboro Pike
Nashville, TN 37215-2715
Tel: 615 292 8606

RICH'S (-MACY'S)
27 stores in three southeastern states
including:
2600 Riverchase Galleria
Birmingham, AL 35244-2394
Tel: 205 985-2600

Also at: 3091 Manchester Expressway
Columbus, GA 31909-6537
Tel: 706 478 2300
700 Haywood Road
Greenville, SC 29607-2781
Tel: 864 297 2020
Tel: 800 241 0488 for customer service
www.richsonline.com

ROUGE BEAUTY BOUTIQUE
539 Rue Dumaine
New Orleans
Louisiana 70116
Tel: 504 525 8686
www.rougebeauty.com

SAKS FIFTH AVENUE
Stores nationwide including:
611 Fifth Avenue
New York, NY 10022
Tel: 212 753 4000
Tel: 877 551 SAKS customer helpline

Also at: 5300 Wisconsin Avenue
Washington DC 20015
Tel: 202 363 2059129
Summit Boulevard
Birmingham, AL 35243
Tel: 205 298 8550

655 Nicollet Mall
Minneapolis, MN 55402
Tel: 612 333 7200

Biltmore Fashion Park
2446 East Camelback Road
Phoenix, AZ 85016
Tel: 602 955 8000

Galleria Mall
2598 East Sunrise Boulevard
Ft. Lauderdale, FL 33304
Tel: 954 563 7600

Pioneer Place Mall
850 SW Fifth Avenue
Portland, OR 97204
Tel: 503 226 3200

1780 Utica Square
Tulsa, OK 74114
Tel: 918 744 0200
www.saksfifthavenue.com

SASSABEE
1849 West North Avenue
Unit C101
Chicago, IL 60622
Tel: 877 828 6073
www.sasabee.com

SEPHORA
Stores nationwide including:
6801 Hollywood Boulevard
Hollywood, CA 90028
Tel: 323 462 6898

Also at: 7007 Friars Road, Suite 314
San Diego, CA 92108
Tel: 619 220 0771

5335 Meadowood Mall Circle
Reno, NV 89502-0560
Tel: 775 826 4561

7400 San Pedro, #104
San Antonio, TX 78216
Tel: 210 541 0979

55 Westfarms Mall
Farmington, CT 06032-2692
Tel: 860 521 7669

2800 W. Big Beaver Road #S 218
Troy, MI 48084
Tel: 248 458 0100

Garden State Plaza
Routes 4 & 17, Space E2
Paramus, NJ 07652
Tel: 201 845 7071

119 E.Franklin St.
Chapel Hill, NC 27514
Tel: 919 932 6777
7101 Democracy Blvd. #2042
Bethesda, MD 20817
Tel: 301 365 9590
Tel: 877-737-4672 for customer service
www.sephora.com

SHU UEMURA BOUTIQUES
WORLDWIDE
For a selection of US stores contact:
121 Greene Street
New York, NY 10012
Tel: 212 979 5500
www.shu-uemura.co.jp

SJAL
330 W. 38th Street, Suite 308
New York, NY 10018
Tel: 212 560 9561
www.isjal.com

TAKASHIMAYA
693 5th Ave at 54th Street
New York, NY 10022-3110
Tel: 212 350 0100

HOME SHOPPING WEBSITES

www.abbeysperfume.com
www.Anyfragrance.com
www.ashford.com
www.ballbeauty.com
www.beautiful4u.com
www.beautifulperfumes.com
www.beautycafe.com
www.beautydeals.net
www.beautydoor.com
www.beautyhabit.com
www.beautyofasite.com
www.beautyrealm.com
www.beautyscene.com
www.centurybeauty.com
www.classyperfumes.com
www.cosmeticmall.com
www.dermadoctor.com
www.dermstore.com
www.diamondbeauty.com
www.discountbeautycenter.com
www.drugstore.com
www.ebay.com
www.ezhaircare.com
www.fabulousfragrances.com
www.folica.com
www.fragrancenet.com
www.gloss.com
www.gotbeauty.com
www.greatskin.com
www.healthandbeautydepot.com
www.HQhair.com
www.laparfumerie.com
www.metrobeauty.com
www.MyPerfume.com
www.onlyfragrances.com
www.parfumsraffy.com
www.perfumeemporium.com
www.perfumehut.com
www.perfumesamerica.com
www.perfumeuniverse.com
www.scentagious.com
www.sephora.com
www.sesto-senso.com
www.shopbodyandsoul.com
www.skinlogic.com
www.skinsite.com
www.skinstore.com
www.spiralhaircase.com
www.strawberrynet.com
www.styleforfree.com/beauty.htm
www.ulta.com
www.visagebeauty.com

REGULATING BODIES, PROFESSIONAL SOCIETIES AND ASSOCIATIONS

THE AMERICAN BOARD OF DERMATOLOGISTS HENRY FORD HEALTH SYSTEM
1 Ford Place
Detroit, MI 48202-3450
Tel: 313 874 1088
www.abderm.org

AMERICAN SOCIETY OF PERFUMERS
PO Box 1551
West Caldwell, NJ 07004
Tel: 201 991 0040
www.perfumers.org

THE COSMETIC, TOILETRY AND FRAGRANCE ASSOCIATION
1101 17th Street NW
Suite 300
Washington DC 20036-4702
Tel: 202 331 1770
www.ctfa.org

PHILIP KINGSLEY TRICHOLOGICAL CLINIC
16 East 53rd Street
New York
NY 10022
Tel: 212 753 9600
www.philipkingsleyny.com

THE SOCIETY OF COSMETIC CHEMISTS (USA)
120 Wall Street #2400
New York, NY 10005-4088
Tel: 212 668 1500
www.scconline.org

www.aad.org
(American Academy of Dermatology)
www.ahbai.org
(American Health and Beauty Aids Institute)
www.consumer.gov
(US Consumer gateway that includes a section on product safety)
www.cosmeticsbusiness.com
www.cosderm.com
(Cosmetic Dermatology)
www.cpsc.gov
(Consumer Product Safety Commission)
www.dermfnd.org
(Dermatology Foundation)
www.fda.gov
(US Food and Drug Administration – for information on cosmetic labelling, safety, ingredients and so on)
www.ftc.gov
(Federal Trade Commission)
www.fragrance.org

PRODUCT REVIEW/TESTING AND INFORMATION WEBSITES

www.beautybuzz.com/scent
www.beautycare.com
www.beautydetective.com
(beauty products watchdog group – online reviews)
www.beautyguru.com
www.beautyproductsearch.com
www.beautywalk.com/rateit
www.bizrate.com (price comparisons between stores, product reviews and store ratings)
www.broadroom.net/daijo/reviews
www.consumerreports.org
www.consumersearch.com
www.cosmeticconnection.com
www.CosmeticIndustry.com
www.cosmeticscop.com/read/reviews.asp
www.ctfa-cir.org (the online version of Cosmetic Ingredient Review)
www.disgruntledhousewife.com/products/beauty.products.html
www.Emakemeup.com
www.epinions.com
www.hairboutique.com/tips/productreviews.htm
www.hair-science.com
www.hintmag.com/beautyduty/beautyduty.php
www.makeupalley.com/product/
www.makeup411.com/new_products.htm
www.mouthshut.com
www.pueblo.gsa.gov (Federal Citizen Information Center, based in Colorado)
www.substance.com/discuss/rate
www.thebeautyreport.net
www.thelipstickpage.com
www.vm.cfsan.fda.gov/~dms/cos-210.html (prohibited ingredients in cosmetics fact sheet)

CANADA

DEPARTMENT STORES, BOUTIQUES AND PHARMACIES

THE BAY
Over 100 stores nationwide including:
Kingsway Garden Mall
109th Street & Princess Elizabeth Avenue
Edmonton, Alberta
T5G 3A6
Tel: 780 479 7100

Also at: 7067 Chbucto Road
Halifax, Nova Scotia
B3L 4R5
Tel: 902 453 1211

Boulevard Centre
4150, rue Jean-Talon Est
Montréal, Québec
H1S 2V4
Tel: 514 728 4571
www.hbc.com/bay

BEAUTYMARK APOTHECARY
1120 Hamilton Street 103
Vancouver, BC V6B 2S2
Tel: 604 642 2294
www.beautymark.ca

BLUSH BEAUTY BAR
1528 17th Avenue SW
Calgary, Alberta
T2T 0C8
Tel: 403 802 4874
www.blushbeautybar.com

THE BODY SHOP
33 Kern Road Don Mills
Ontario M3B 1S9
Tel: 416 441 3202
www.thebodyshop.com

HELENA RUBINSTEIN
2115 rue Crescent
Montréal, Québec CODE
Tel: 514 335 8000 for stockists

HOLT RENFREW
Stores nationwide including:
50 Bloor Street West
Toronto, Ontario
M4W1A1
Tel: 416 922 2333

Also at: 1300 Sherbrooke Street West
Montreal, Quebec
H3G1H9
Tel: 514 842 5111

633 Granville Street
Vancouver, BC
V7Y1E4
Tel: 866 465 8736 for mail order
www.holtrenfrew.com

ICE
163 Cumberland
Toronto, Ontario
ON M5R1A2
Tel: 416 964 6751

LOLA & EMILY
3475 St Laurent Blvd
Montréal, Québec
H2X 2T6
Tel: 514 288 7598
www.lolaandemily.com

LONDON DRUGS LTD
2032 Lonsdale
North Vancouver, BC
V7M 2K5
Tel: 604 448 4805

MAISON FRAGRANCE
The Home of Perfumes
and Beauty
9610-F Ignace street
Brossard, Québec
J4Y 2R4
Tel: 800 761 1196
or 450 444 1808
www.maisonfragrance.com

OGILVY
1307 Ste-Catherine West
Montreal, QC
H3G1P7
Tel: 514 842 7711

OUTER LAYER
430 Bloor Street West
Toronto, Ontario
CODE
Tel: 416 324 8333

Also at: 577 Queen Street West
Toronto, Ontario
Tel: 416 869 9889
www.outerlayer.ca

PIR COSMETICS
25 Bellair Street
Toronto, Ontario
CODE
Tel: 416 513 1603
www.theartofbeauty.com

RUBIES BEAUTY BAR
715 Queen Street West
Toronto, Ontario
M6J 1E6
Tel: 416 601 6789
www.rubiesbeautybar.com

SHIFEON
1156 Robson Street
Vancouver, BC
V6E 1B2
Tel: 888 291 6027 or 604 688 3291
www.perfumewww.com

SHU UEMURA
1361 Greene Avenue
Montréal, Québec
CODE
Tel: 514 932 1444

Also at: 25 Bellair Street
Toronto, Ontario
Tel: 416 513 1603

WANTSTIL BOUTIQUE
231 St. Paul West
Montréal, Québec
H2A 2A2
Tel: 514 499 8549

**A WORLD OF PERFUMES
AND COSMETICS STORE**
3-5420 Dundee Street
Vancouver, BC
V5R 5Y7
Tel: 604 430 6372
www.a-world-of-perfumes-
cosmetics.com

REGULATING
BODIES,
PROFESSIONAL
SOCIETIES AND
ASSOCIATIONS

**CANADIAN CONSUMER
SPECIALTY PRODUCTS
ASSOCIATION**
56 Sparks St #500
Ottawa K1P 5A9
Tel: 613 232 6616

**CANADIAN COSMETIC,
TOILETRY AND FRAGRANCE
ASSOCIATION**
420 Britannia Road East #102
Mississauga L4Z 3L5
Tel: 905-890-5161
www.cctfa.ca

AUSTRALIA

DEPARTMENT
STORES, BOUTIQUES
AND PHARMACIES

BETTERSKIN
Shop 3
105 Miller street
North Sydney, NSW 2060
Tel: 1300 133 631
www.betterskin.com.au

BEYOND BEAUTY
2/46 Gayford Street
Aspley QLD 4024
Tel: 07 3263 9915 or 07 3263 5755

THE BODY ORCHARD
33 Vincent Street
Daylesford, Victoria 3460
Tel: 03 5348 4111

THE BODY SHOP AUSTRALIA
Adidem Pty Ltd
Wellington and Jacksons Road
Mulgrave
Melbourne, Victoria 3170
Tel: 03 9565 0500
www.thebodyshop.com.au

THE COMPLETE BASKET CASE
61 Burns Road
Springwood NSW 2777
Tel: 1300 733 933
Tel: 02 4751 1642 for international
enquiries
www.thebasketcase.com.au

DIMI'S BODY AND SOUL
Shop 1
1 Bond St
Hurstville 2220
Tel: 02 9579 4455
www.dimisbodyandsoul.com

FRENDLIES CHEMISTS
136 Rokeby Rd
Subiaco, WA 6008
Tel: 08 9381 1468
www.friendliessubiaco.com

HE & HER PERFUMERY
Shop 14
Rundle Arcade
Adelaide SA CODE
Tel: 08 212 5239

DAVID JONES
Elizabeth Street
Sydney, NSW 2000
Tel : 09 266 5544
Tel: 1300 300 110 for general
enquiries

Also at: Rundall Mall
Adelaide, SA
Tel: 08 305 3000

310 Bourke Street
Melbourne, VIC 3001
Tel: 3 9643 2222
Queen Street Mall
Queen Street
Brisbane, QLD 4000
Tel: 7 3243 9000
www.davidjones.com.au

MECCA COSMETICS
Shop 56 Oxford Street
Paddington, NSW 0000
Tel: 02 9361 4488

Also at: South Yarra
Shop 1, 166 Toorak Road
Victoria 3141
Tel: 03 9827 8711

Bayview Terrace,
Claremont
Perth, Western Australia
Tel: 08 9286 2477
www.meccacosmetica.com.au

MYER
Myer Adelaide
22 Rundall Mall
Adelaide, SA CODE
Tel: 08 8205 9111
www.myer.com.au

Also at: Myer Centre
Queen St
Brisbane, QLD 4000
Tel: 07 3232 0121

Forest Chase
Wellington St
Perth, WA 6000
Tel: 08 9221 3444

314-366 Bourke St
Melbourne, VIC 3000
Tel: 03 9661 1111

GRACE BROS
Penrith Plaza
Penrith NSW 2750
Tel: 02 4721 4331
www.gracebros.com.au

NATIONAL PHARMACIES
52 Gawler Place
Adelaide, SA 5000
Tel: 08 223 0300

Also at: 235 Queen Street
Melbourne Victoria 3000
Tel: 03 9642 2555

31 Windsor Road
Kellyville, NSW 2155
Tel: 02 9629 140
www.nationalpharmacies.com.au

THE PAINTED PONY
784 Glenferrie Road
Hawthorn 3122
Tel: 03 9818 1803
www.thepaintedpony.com.au

PETERS OF KENSINGTON
57 Anzac Parade Kensington
Sydney CODE
Tel: 02 9662 1099
www.petersofkensington.com.au

**JOHN PRITCHARD
INTERNATIONAL**
327-331 Main Street
Mornington,
Victoria 3931
Tel: 1300 300 954

PHYTOLOGY
222 Given Tce
Paddington,
Queensland 4064
Tel: 07 3369 7770
www.phytology.com.au

**SCENT BODY
AND BATH**
147 Maling Road
Canterbury, CODE
Tel: 03 9836 4766

SHOP 4
74 Doncaster Road
North Balwyn 3104
Tel: 03 9859 7666

TERRY WHITE CHEMISTS
Shop 1, Annandale Shopping Centre
Crn University Road & MacArthur Drive
Annandale 4814
Tel: 07 4725 1112

Also at: 372 Fitzgerald Street
North Perth, 6006
Tel: 08 9328 5762

Level E The Myer Centre
Queen St
Brisbane QLD 4000 Australia
Tel: 07 3221 3416
www.terrywhitechemists.com.au

TEMPLE EMPORIUM
444 Chapel Street
South Yarra
Victoria 3141
Tel: 03 9827 2770

URBAN ATTITUDE
152 Auckland Street
St Kilda Victoria CODE
Tel: 03 9525 5977
also at Federation Square in Melbourne
Tel: 9663 6680
www.urbanattitude.com.au

HOME SHOPPING WEBSITES

www.adorebeauty.com.au
www.beautysupplies.com.au
www.buyquick.com.au
www.cbeauty.com.au
www.ebay.com.au
www.efragrance.com.au
www.ellarouge.com.au
www.healthbasket.com.au
www.mjhealthandbeauty.com.au
www.mysuperdeals.com.au
www.oakhillnailspa.com.au
www.pharmacyonline.com.au
www.priceattack.com.au
www.rigall.com.au
www.shoppersdirect.com.au
www.signature-perfumes.com.au
www.vitaminsaustralia.com.au
www.wishlist.com.au

REGULATING BODIES, PROFESSIONAL SOCIETIES AND ASSOCIATIONS

THE AUSTRALASIAN COLLEGE OF DERMATOLOGISTS
PO Box B65
Boronia Park, NSW 2111
Tel: 02 9879 6177
www.dermcoll.asn.au

AUSTRALIAN CONSUMERS' ASSOCIATION
57 Carrington Road
Marrickville, NSW 2204
Tel: 02 9577 3399

AUSTRALIAN MEDICAL ASSOCIATION
42 Macquarie Street
Barton, ACT 2600
and
PO Box E115
Kingston, ACT 2604
Tel: 02 6270 5400

INTERNATIONAL ASSOCIATION OF TRICHOLOGISTS
185 Elizabeth Street, Suite 919
Sydney, NSW 2000
TEL: 02 9267 1384
www.virtualhaircare.com.au/virtual%2
0salon/trichology/trich.html

TRI INSTITUTE OF TRICHOLOGY
PO Box 172
Paddington, Queensland 4064
Tel: 0500 888 859
www.trihaircare.com.au

PRODUCT REVIEW/TESTING AND INFORMATION WEBSITES WWW.ACCC.GOV.AU (AUSTRALIAN COMPETITION AND CONSUMER COMMISSION)
www.austrade.gov.au (Australian Trade Commission)
www.cleoninene.com.au
www.Choice.com.au (Choice Online)

BRAND DIRECTORY

ALEXANDER MCQUEEN
www.alexandermcqueen.net
Tel: 020 7278 4333 (UK)

ALMAY
www.almay.com

AMANDA LACEY
Tel: 020 7370 4410 (UK)

ANDREW COLLINGE
www.andrewcollinge.com
Tel: 0151 709 5942 (UK)

ANNA SUI
www.annasuibeauty.com
Tel: 020 7499 4420 (UK); 212 941 8406
(USA); 02 9663 4277 (Australia)

ANNICK GOUTAL
www.annickgoutal.nl
Tel: 020 7734 1234 (UK)

ANTONIA'S FLOWERS
www.antoniasflowers.com
Tel: 0870 169 9999 (UK); 800 332 5558
(USA); 03 9827 3844 (Australia)

AUSSIE
www.aussie.com

AVEDA
www.aveda.com
Tel: 020 7297 6350 (UK); 866 823 1425
(USA); 03 9419 3555 (Australia)

AVON
www.avon.com
Tel: 0845 601 4040 (UK); 800 500 2866
(USA); 514 695 3371 (Canada);
02 9936 7555 (Australia)

AWAKE
www.awakecosmetics.com

BABYLISS
www.babyliss.com

BALENCIAGA FRAGRANCES
www.balenciaga.com
Tel: 212 279 4440 (US)

BARRY M
www.barrym.com
Tel: 020 8349 2992 (UK)

BECCA COSMETICS
www.beccacosmetics.com

BENEFIT
www.benefitcosmetic.com
Tel: 09011 130 001 (UK);
800 781 2336 (USA)

BIOELEMENTS
www.bioelements.com
Tel: 800 533 3064 (USA)

BIORE
www.biore.com
Tel: 888 BIORE 11 (USA)

BIOTHERM
www.biotherm.com
www.us.biotherm.com

BLACK LIKE ME
www.blacklikeme.co.za
Tel: 27 11 541 0100 (South Africa)

BLISS SPA
www.blissworld.com
Tel: 020 7584 3888 (UK);
212 219 8970 (USA)

BLOOM COSMETICS
www.bloomcosmetics.com
Tel: 020 8735 2882 (UK)

BOBBI BROWN ESSENTIALS
www.bobbibrowncosmetics.com
Tel: 01730 232 566 / 0800 5070 8090
(UK); 212 980 7040 (USA);
416 413 5250 (Canada);
02 9381 1390 (Australia)

THE BODY SHOP
www.thebodyshop.com
Tel: 01903 731500 (UK); 919 554 4900
(USA); 416 441 3202 (Canada);
03 9565 0500 (Australia)

BORGHESE
www.borghese.com
Tel: 01273 408 800 (UK);
1 866 BORGHESE (USA)

BOURJOIS
www.bourjois.com
Tel: 0800 269 8386 (UK)

BRAUN
www.braun.com
Tel: 0800 7837010 (UK); 800 272 8611
(USA); 1300 363937 (Australia)

BRENDA CHRISTIAN
www.brendachristian.safeserver.com
Tel: 800 759 8498 (US)

BULGARI
www.bulgari.com

BUMBLE AND BUMBLE
www.bumbleandbumble.com
Tel: 01768 895 505 /
020 7299 4999 (UK)

BURBERRY
www.burberry.com

BURT'S BEES
www.burtsbees.com

CACHAREL
www.cacharel.com

CALVIN KLEIN
Tel: 020 7361 4400 (UK);
800 223 6808 (USA);
905 829 5150 (Canada);
02 9869 6100 (Australia)

CARGO COSMETICS
www.cargocosmetics.com

CARON
www.parfums-caron.com
Tel: 020 7730 1234 (UK)

CARTIER
www.cartier.com
Tel: 020 7408 5700 (UK);
415 397 3180 (USA);
416 413 4929 (Canada);
03 9650 2602 (Australia)

CAUDALIE
www.caudalie.com

CHANEL
www.chanel.com
Tel: 020 7493 3836 (UK);
800 550 0005 (USA)

CHARLES WORTHINGTON
www.cwlondon.com
Tel: 020 7636 4686 (UK)

CHLOE
www.chloe.com
Tel: 020 7823 5348 (UK);
212 717 8220 (USA)

CHRISTIAN DIOR
www.dior.com
Tel: 01932 233902 (UK);
800 929 DIOR (USA)

CIRCAROMA
www.circaroma.com
Tel: 020 7249 9502 (UK)

CITRE SHINE
www.citreshine.com

CLARINS
www.clarins.com
Tel: 020 7307 6700 (UK)

CLAIROL
www.clairol.com
Tel: 0800 181184 (UK); 800 252 4765
(USA); 800 252 4765 (Canada);
800 226 525 (Australia)

CLAIROL HERBAL ESSENCES
www.herbalessences.com

CLE DE PEAU BEAUTE
www.cledepeau.com

CLINIQUE
www.clinique.com
Tel: 01730 232 566 (UK);
212 572 3800 (USA)

COSMETICS A LA CARTE LTD
www.cosmeticsalacarte.com
Tel: 020 7622 2318 (UK)

CRABTREE AND EVELYN
www.crabtree-evelyn.com
Tel: 020 7361 0499 / 01235 864 824;
800 272 2873 (USA)

CREATIVE NAIL DESIGN
www.creativenail.com

CREED
www.creedfragrances.com
Tel: 020 7630 9400 (UK)

DANIEL FIELD
www.danielfield.com

DANIEL GALVIN
www.daniel-gavin.co.uk
Tel: 020 7486 9661

DARPHIN
www.darphin.fr
Tel: 020 8847 18777 (UK)

DECLEOR
www.decleor.com
Tel: 020 7402 9474 (UK); 800 722 2219
(USA); 029 557 1177 (Australia);
450 963 5096 (Canada)

DENMAN
www.denmanbrush.com
Tel: 0800 262 509 (UK); 800 848 6866
(USA); 514 345 0949 (Canada);
612 9557 2071 (Australia)

DERMALOGICA
www.dermalogica.com
Tel: 0800 591818 (UK)

DIPTYQUE
www.diptyque.tm.fr

**DOCTOR'S DERMALOGIC
FORMULA**
www.ddfskin.com

DR HAUSCHKA
www.drhauschka.com
Tel: 01386 792 642 (UK); 800 247 9907
(USA); 02 9818 6119 (Australia)

DOLCE & GABBANA
www.dolcegabbana.it

DUWOP
www.duwoponline.com

ELEMIS LTD
www.elemis.com
Tel: 020 8954 8033 (UK); 866
ELEMISSPA (USA); 800 423 5293
(Canada); 02 9238 0000 (Australia)

ELIZABETH ARDEN
www.elizabetharden.com
Tel: 020 7574 2700 (UK);
212 261 1000 (USA)

E'SPA
www.espaonline.com
Tel: 01252 742800 (UK)

ESTEE LAUDER
www.esteelauder.com
Tel: 01730 232 566 (UK); 212 572 4433
(USA); 416 413 5268 (Canada);
02 9381 1344 (Australia)

ETRO
www.etro.com
Tel: 020 7495 5767 (UK);
212 317 9096 (USA)

EVE LOM
www.evelom.com
Tel: 020 8661 7991 / 0870 169 9999
(UK); 888 334 FACE (USA)

EYEKO
www.eyebeautyusa.com
Tel: 020 7734 9090 (UK);
800 89 EYEKO (USA)

FARMACIA
www.farmacia.co.uk
Tel: 020 7404 8808 (UK)

FASHION FAIR
www.fashionfaircosmetics.com

FREDERIC FEKKAI
www.fredericfekai.com

FRESH
www.fresh.com
Tel: 800 FRESH 209 (USA)

FUDGE
www.fudge.com
Tel: 01282 683 100 (UK); 818 993 8343
/ 888 FUD GEUS (USA)

GARNIER
www.garnierbeautybar.com
www.garnierusa.com
Tel: 0845 399 0104 (UK); 514 535 800
(Canada); 03 9272 222 (Australia)

GATINEAU
Tel: 0800 731 5805 (UK)

GIORGIO ARMANI
www.giorgioarmani.com
Tel: 212 988 9191 (USA);
866 276 2640 (Canada)

GIVENCHY
www.givenchy.com
Tel: 020 7730 1234 (UK)

GUCCI
www.gucci.com

GUERLAIN
www.guerlain.com
Tel: 020 7730 1234 / 01932 233 874
(UK); 800 815 7720 (USA);
514 363 0432 (Canada)

GUINOT
www.guinotusa.com
Tel: 01344 873 123 (UK);
800 444 6621 (USA)

HARD CANDY
www.hardcandy.com
Tel: 949 515 1250 (USA)

HEALTHY SEXY HAIR CONCEPTS
www.cutndry.com
Tel: 888 344 8484 (US)

HELENA RUBINSTEIN
www.helenarubinstein.com
Tel: 020 8762 4040 (UK); 212 818 1500
(USA); 514 335 8000 (Canada)

HELMUT LANG
www.helmutlang.com
Tel: 866 81HLANG (USA)

HERMES
www.hermes.com
Tel: 020 7499 8856 (UK); 800 441 4488
(USA); 604 681 9965 (Canada); 03
9654 5571 (Australia)

HUGO BOSS
www.hugo.com

ICE HAIR
www.icehair.com

IMAN COSMETICS
www.i-iman.com
Tel: 800 366 4626 (USA)

**JANE IREDALE MINERAL
COSMETICS**
www.janeiredale.com
Tel: 020 8450 7111 (UK); 800 817 5665
(USA); 800 661 7125 (Canada);
800 66 4455 (Australia)

**JEAN-PAUL GAULTIER
FRAGRANCES**
www.jeanpaul-gaultier.com

JERGENS
www.jergens.com

JESSICA
www.jessicacosmetics.com

JING JANG
www.jingjang.com
Tel: 888 458 3520 (USA)

J F LAZARTIGUE
www.jflazartigue.com
Tel: 800 359 9345 (USA)

JO HANSFORD
www.johansford.com

JO MALONE
www.jomalone.com
Tel: 020 7730 2100 / 020 7720 0202
(UK); 212 673 2220 (USA);
416 922 2333 (Canada)

JOHN FRIEDA
www.johnfrieda.com
Tel: 800 521 3189 (USA); 416 922 2333
(Canada); 03 9371 8817 (Australia)

JOICO
www.joico.com
Tel: 818 968 6111 / 800 44J OICO (USA)

JOOP!
www.joop.com

JURLIQUE
www.jurlique.com
Tel: 020 8841 6644 (UK); 800 854 1110
(USA); 618 8391 0577 (Australia)

JUVENA
www.juvena.ch
Tel: 561 655 7816 (USA); 450 465 4300
(Canada); 02 9888 0600 (Australia)

KANEBO
www.kanebo.com
Tel: 01635 46362 (UK);
866 271 6815 (USA)

KENT
www.kentbrushes.com
Tel: 01442 23 26 23 (UK)

KENZO
www.kenzo.com

KERASTASE
www.kerastase.com

KIEHL'S
www.kiehls.com
Tel: 020 7240 2411 (UK); 800 KIEHLS 2
/ 800 543 4572 (USA)

KMS
www.kmshaircare.com

KORRES
www.korres.com

LABORATOIRE REMEDE
www.remede.com

LACOSTE FRAGRANCES
www.lacoste.com

L'ARTISAN PARFUMEUR
www.artisanparfumeur.com
Tel: 020 7352 4196 (UK)

L'ANZA
www.lanza.com

LA PRAIRIE
www.laprairie.com
Tel: 020 8398 5300 (UK);
800 821 5718 (USA);
02 9888 6333 (Australia)

LANCASTER
www.lancaster-beauty.com

LANCOME
www.lancome.com
Tel: 020 8762 4040 (UK);
800 LANCOME (USA)

LAURA BIAGIOTTI
www.laurabiagiotti.com

LAURA MERCIER
www.lauramercier.com
Tel: 0870 169 9999 (UK);
888 MERCIER (USA)

LIZ COLLINGE
www.lizcollingecosmetics.com
Tel: 0115 949 4499 (UK)

LIZ EARLE
www.lizearle.net
Tel: 01983 813913 (UK)

L'OCCITANE
www.loccitane.com
Tel: 020 7907 0300 / 020 7907 0301
(UK); 02 8339 0111 (Australia)

LOLA
www. Lolacosmetics.com
Tel: 866 BUY LOLA (US)

LORAC
www.loraccosmetics.com
Tel: 800 845 0705 (USA)

L'OREAL
www.lorealparis.com
Tel: 0845 399 1959 (UK);
888 456 7325 (Canada)

MAC COSMETICS
www.maccosmetics.com
Tel: 020 7534 9222 (UK); 800 387 6707
(USA); 416 979 2171 (Canada); 03
9661 3909 / 02 9238 9141 (Australia)

MAKE UP FOR EVER
www.makeupforever.com
Tel: 020 7529 5690 (UK); 212 941 9337
(USA); 514 288 4445 (Canada);
02 9695 4829 (Australia)

MARC JACOBS
www.marcjacobs.com
Tel: 020 7563 8800 (UK);
212 343 1490 (USA)

MARIO BADESCU
www.mariobadescu.com
Tel: 212 758 1065 (US)

MARTHA HILL
www.marthahill.com
Tel: 0800 980 6664 (UK)

MASON PEARSON BROS LTD
www.masonpearson.com
Tel: 020 7491 2613 (UK); 516 599 1176
(USA); 03 9587 4700 (Australia)

MATIS
www.matis-uk.com
Tel: 01322 290101 (UK)

MATRIX
www.matrixbeautiful.com
Tel: 888 777 6396 (USA)

MAX FACTOR
www.maxfactor.com
Tel: 0800 169 1302 (UK);
03 9548 8944 (Australia)

MAYBELLINE
www.maybelline.com
Tel: 0845 399 0304 (UK); 800 944 0730
(USA); 514 335 8000 (Canada);
613 9272 222 (Australia)

MICHAEL KORS
www.kors.com
Tel: 020 7235 5000 (UK);
800 375 0417 (USA)

MILLER HARRIS
www.millerharris.com
Tel: 020 7221 1545 (UK)

MOLTON BROWN COSMETICS
www.moltonbrown.com
Tel: 020 7499 6474 /
020 7625 6550 (UK)

MOP (MODERN ORGANIC PRODUCTS)
www.mopproducts.com
Tel: 01282 613413 (UK);
866 699 4667 (USA)

MORPHY RICHARDS
www.morphyrichards.co.uk
Tel: 08450 777700 (UK)

MOSCHINO FRAGRANCES
www.moschino.com

MURAD
www.murad.com
Tel: 888 99 MURAD (USA)

NAILTIQUES COSMETIC CORPORATION
www.nailtiques.com
Tel: 800 272 0054 /
305 378 0740 (USA)

NARS
www.narscosmetics.com
Tel: 020 7517 9497 (UK);
888 903 6277 (USA)

NASCENT
www.nascentorganic.com
Tel: 45 39 15 77 22 (Denmark)

NEAL'S YARD REMEDIES
www.nealsyardremedies.com
Tel: 020 7379 7222 / 0161 831 7875
(UK); 888 697 4451 (USA);
02 9233 5404 (Australia)

NEXXUS
www.nexxusproducts.com

NICKY CLARKE
www.nickyclarke.co.uk

NIVEA
www.nivea.com
Tel: 0800 616 977 (UK)

NEUTROGENA
www.neutrogena.com
Tel: 01628 822 2222 (UK);
800 582 4048 (USA)

NICKY CLARKE
www.nickyclarke.com

NINA RICCI
www.ninaricci.com
Tel: 020 7290 6716 (UK); 212 980 9620
(USA); 416 620 3979 (Canada)

NUXE
www. Nuxe.com
Tel: 01932 827060 (UK);
450 963 5096 (US);
450 433 8918 (Canada)

OLAY
www.olay.com
Tel: 0800 917 7197 (UK);
800 028 280 (Australia)

OLE HENRIKSEN
www.olefacebody.com
Tel: 310 854 7700 (USA)

OPI NAILS
www.opi.com
Tel: 020 8868 3400 (UK); 800 341 9999
(USA); 02 9486 3211 (Australia)

ORLANE
www.orlaneparis.com

ORIGINS
www.origins.com
Tel: 0800 731 4039 (UK);
800 723 7310 (USA);
613 721 4537 (Canada);
02 9238 9111 (Australia)

OSCAR DE LA RENTA
www.oscardelarenta.com

PACO RABANNE
www.pacorabanne.com

PASSPORT
www.passportcosmetics.com

PANTENE
www.pantene.com

PAUL MITCHELL
www.paulmitchell.com

PAUL SMITH
www.paulsmith.co.uk

PAULA DORF
www.pauladorf.com

PENHALIGON'S
www.penhaligons.co.uk
Tel: 0800 716108 / 0207 747 7899
(UK); 877 736 4254 (USA)

PHILIP B
www.philipb.com

PHILOSOPHY
www.philosophy.com
Tel: 0845 070 8090 (UK)

PHYTOLOGY
www.phytology.com.au
Tel: 02 3369 7770 (Australia)

PHYTOMER
www.phytomer.com

PHYSICIAN'S FORMULA
www.physiciansformula.com

PIXI
www.pixibeauty.com
Tel: 020 7287 7211 (UK)

PONDS
www.ponds.com
Tel: 800 743 8640 (USA)

POUT
www.pout.co.uk
Tel: 020 7379 0379 (UK)

PRADA
www.prada.com
Tel: 020 7235 0008 (UK)

PRESCRIPTIVES
www.gloss.com/px
Tel: 01730 232 566 (UK);
212 572 4400 (USA)

PRETTY PRETTY COSMETICS
www.pretty2.com
Tel: 866 773 8892 (USA)

PUPA
www.pupa.it

RALPH LAUREN
www.polo.com
Tel: 020 7535 4600 (UK);
888 475 7674 (USA);
514 288 3988 (Canada);
0 2 9267 1630 / 03 9654 0374 (Australia)

REDKEN
www.redken.com
Tel: 0800 44 880 (UK); 800 REDKEN 8
(USA); 888 REDKEN 0 (Canada)

REMINGTON
www.remington-products.com
Tel: 0800 212 438 (UK); 800 736 4648
(USA); 1 800 623 118 (Australia)

REN
www.ren.ltd.uk
Tel: 020 7935 2323 (UK)

REVLON (AND ALMAY)
www.revlon.com
Tel: 0800 085 2716 (UK); 800 473 8566
(USA); 800 025 488 (Australia)

RIMMEL
www.rimmellondon.com
Tel: 020 8971 1300 (UK)

ROBERTO CAVALLI
www.robertocavalli.net
Tel: 212 3085566 (USA)

ROC
www.roc.com

ST TROPEZ
www.sttropeztan.com
Tel: 0115 9221 462 (UK);
661 775 6900 (USA)

SALLY HANSEN
www.sallyhansen.com

SCHWARZKOPF
www.schwarzkopf.com
Tel: 01296 314 000 (UK); 800 022 219
(USA); 800 022 219 (Australia)

SCREEN FACE
www.screenface.com
Tel: 020 7836 3955 (UK)

SEBASTIAN
www.sebastian-intl.com
Tel: 800 829 7322 (USA)

SEPHORA
www.sephora.com
Tel: 01923 244 918 (UK);
877 737 4672 (USA)

SHISEIDO
www.shiseido.co.uk
Tel: 020 7836 5588 (UK);
800 423 5339 (USA)

SHU UEMURA
www.shu-uemura.co.jp
Tel: 020 7379 6627 (UK); 212 979 5500
(USA); 416 513 1603 (Canada)

SISLEY
www.sisley-cosmetics.com
Tel: 0207 491 2722 (UK); 214 528 8006
/ 214 528 5661 (USA); 416 922 2333 /
416 960 5477 (Canada);
02 9282 9977 (Australia)

SJAL
www.isjal.com
Tel: 212 560 9561 (USA)

SK-II
www.sk2.com

SMASHBOX
www.smashbox.com

SPACE NK
www.spacenk.co.uk
Tel: 020 7299 4999 / 0870 169 9999 (UK)

SPORNETTE BRUSHES
www.spornette.com
Tel: 800 323 6449 (USA)

STILA
www.stilacosmetics.com
Tel: 01730 232 566 (UK); 877 565 1299
(USA); 416 413 5250 (Canada);
02 9381 1200 (Australia)

TARTE
www.tartecosmetics.com
Tel: 212 247 1100 (USA)

TE TAO
www.tetao.com

TERAX HAIR
www.teraxhaircare.com
Tel: 020 7229 0563 (UK);
315 458 2290 (USA)

THALGO
www.thalgo.co.uk
Tel: 0800 146041 (UK)

THIERRY MUGLER PARFUMS
www.thierrymugler.com
Tel: 020 7307 6700 (UK); 212 758 0400
(USA); 514 745 0190 (Canada);
02 9663 4277 (Australia)

THREE CUSTOM COLOR
www.threecustom.com
Tel: 888 262 7714 (USA)

TIGI
www.tigihaircare.com
Tel: 020 8388 1300 / 0870 3300 955
(UK); 972 931 1567 (USA);
02 9439 9666 (Australia)

TISSERAND
www.tisserand.com
Tel: 01273 325666 (UK)

TOCCA
www.tocca.com
Tel: 212 929 7122 (USA)

TOMMY HILFIGER
www.tommy.com
Tel: 01730 232566 (UK);
800 866 6922 / 877 866 6922 (USA)

TONY AND TINA
www.tonytina.com
Tel: 888 TONYTINA /
212 226 3992 (USA)

TONI AND GUY
www.toniandguy.com
Tel: 0800 731 2396 (UK)

TOO FACED
www.toofaced.com

TREVOR SORBIE
www.trevorsorbie.com
Tel: 01372 375 235 (UK)

ST TROPEZ
www.sttropeztan.com
Tel: 0115 922 1462 (UK);
661 775 6900 (USA)

TWEEZERMAN
www.tweezerman.com
Tel: 888 647 7377 (USA)

UMBERTO GIANNINI
www.umbertogiannini.com
Tel: 01384 444771 (UK)

URBAN DECAY
www.urbandecay.com
Tel: 800 784 URBAN /
949 631 4504 (USA)

VAN CLEEF & ARPELS
www.vca-parfums.com
Tel: 212 715 7333 (USA)

VALENTINO
www.valentino.it
Tel: 020 7535 5855 (UK)

VERA WANG FRAGRANCES
www.verawang.com

VIDAL SASSOON
www.vidalsassoon.com
Tel: 0800 072 1661 (UK)

VINCENT LONGO
www.vincentlongo.com
Tel: 877 LONGO 99 /
305 778 4575 (USA)

VIVIENNE WESTWOOD
www.viviennewestwood.com

VICHY
www.vichy.com

WELEDA
www.weleda.com
Tel: 0115 9448200 (UK); 800 241 1030
(USA); 03 9723 7278 (Australia)

WELLA
www.wella.com
Tel: 01256 320202 (UK); 818 999 5112
(USA); 905 568 2494 (Canada);
02 9888 766 5 (Australia)

YVES SAINT LAURENT
www.ysl.com
Tel: 01444 255 700 (UK);
212 753 4000 (USA)

ZIRH
www.zirh.com
Tel: 800 295 8877 /
212 813 2100 (USA)

PICTURE CREDITS

The publishers would like to thank the following sources for their kind permission to reproduce the pictures in this book:page 1 © Carlton Books/Patrice De Villiers; page 2 Courtesy Dowal Walker PR; page 4 Courtesy Prada PR; page 6 © Carlton Books; page 7 Courtesy La Prairie PR; page 10 Courtesy Stila Cosmetics PR; page 11 Courtesy YSL Beauté; page 12 Courtesy Elizabeth Arden PR; page 14 Courtesy Estée Lauder PR; page 15 Courtesy Clinique PR; page 16 © Carlton Books; page 17 © Carlton Books; page 18 © Carlton Books/Patrice De Villiers; page 22 Courtesy Almay PR; page 23 Estée Lauder PR; page 25 © Carlton Books/Patrice De Villiers; page 26 Courtesy Wizard PR; page 27 Courtesy Estée Lauder PR; page 28 Courtesy Purple PR; page 29 Courtesy Purple PR; page 30 Courtesy Laura Mercier PR; page 31 © Carlton Books/Patrice De Villiers; page 32 Courtesy Wizard PR.

Every effort has been made to acknowledge correctly and contact the source and/or copyright holder of each picture, and Carlton Books Limited apologizes for any un-intentional errors or omissions, which will be corrected in future editions of this book.

AUTHOR ACKNOWLEDGEMENTS

Special thanks go to Anne Carullow, Dominique Szabo and Dr Daniel Maes at Estée Lauder, and Philip Kingsley, Wendy Lewis, Amanda Lacey, Eve Lom, Luci Rogers, Ruby Hammer and Laura Mercier. I would also like to thank the Cosmetic, Toiletry and Perfumery Association and the Soil Association, as well as the panel of women who made the book possible by testing over 1000 products. Thanks, too, to my editor, Lisa Dyer, and editorial manager, Judith More, at Carlton Books.

The publishers would like to thank Claire Musters and Sarah Sears for the directory.